BE YOUR OWN PT

A Proven 10-Week Weight Training & Diet Program For Your Self-Transformation

By Marc McLean

Copyright 2020 Marc McLean

All rights reserved

Author's Legal Disclaimer

This book is solely for informational and educational purposes and is not medical advice. Please consult a medical or health professional before you begin any new exercise, nutrition or supplementation program, or if you have questions about your health.

Always put safety first when lifting weights in the gym. Any use of the information within this book is at the reader's discretion and risk.

The author cannot be held responsible for any loss, claim or damage arising out of the use, or misuse, of the suggestions made, the failure to take medical advice, or for any related material from third party sources.

No part of this publication shall be reproduced, transmitted, or sold in any form without the prior written consent of the author.

All trademarks and registered trademarks appearing in this digital book are the property of their respective owners.

Contents

Introduction 1

PART ONE: PREPARATION

Chapter 1: PT vs Yourself 7

Chapter 2: Weight Training // Intermittent Fasting // Accountability 13

Chapter 3: Various Fitness Goals, One Approach 31

PART TWO: THE PROGRAMME

Chapter 4: Mastering The Compounds (Week 1) 46

Chapter 5: Intermittent Fasting (Week 2) 58

Chapter 6: The Three Set Shocker (Week 3) 72

Chapter 7: Time For Some Personal Bests (Week 4) 78

Chapter 8: Isolation Exercises For Muscle Definition (Week 5) 84

Chapter 9: Drop Sets (Week 6) 90

Chapter 10: Creating A Stronger Self Image (Week 7) 96

Chapter 11: It's Time To Burn (Week 8) 105

Chapter 12: Rising To A Whole New Level (Week 9) 112

Chapter 13: The Final Push...And Celebrations (Week 10) 118

PART THREE: SUCCESS STORIES

Chapter 14: From A 310lbs Mountain Of Flab…To A Rock Solid Gym Machine...124

Chapter 15: Athlete Finds The Strength To Get Back To The Top 131

Chapter 16: A Woman's Decades-Long Fitness Search Is Over ..141

Chapter 17: Muscle & Strength Without A Military Style Approach...148

Chapter 18: Weight Training Has Got Me Back On Track 154

Chapter 19: I Wanted To Be A Fitter And Healthier Dad 158

Bonus Chapter: Supplements 167

Conclusion 177

About The Author 182

EXERCISES INDEX..185

Introduction

Finding a gym program that actually delivers clear results isn't the only problem you're faced with these days.

No, an even bigger issue is discovering an approach to weight training that you enjoy AND a diet that can be maintained in the long term.

Otherwise, you get bored, frustrated, willpower runs out…and then it's back to looking for the next best workout trend (while munching on a 20-inch pizza just to emotionally get over the latest fitness failure).

Forget all that. You don't have to trudge through mind-numbing, repetitive gym workouts, or spend a fortune on personal trainers, or torture yourself with strict diet plans that you hate.

In fact, it can – and should – be the complete opposite.

How does an exciting workout program where you continually challenge yourself and look forward to every gym session sound?

How about a well-structured set-up that's centered around you smashing personal bests and achieving what you never thought was possible in the gym?

And do you like the idea of not only lifting weights in the most effective way to become strong and fit as hell, but also complementing it with a healthy diet approach that doesn't ban all your favourite foods and you don't struggle to maintain either?

You've found it. In this book, I'm about to lay out, step-by-step, my unique 10-week weight training and diet program. It's a proven approach I've refined over the past 10 years or so – and is a program I've already used to great effect when coaching men and women all over the world.

You see, I run a 10-week online weight training and diet course called 'Be Your Own PT'.

DON'T PANIC – I'm not going to try to sell you onto it, or sell you anything at all in this book. Promise.

I only open up the online course 3-4 times per year, and it's restricted to just 10-15 people at a time because I want to give each person the best coaching I can throughout the 10-week duration.

That's exactly why I'm now making the Be Your Own PT program available in book format – so that all the golden information I've learned over the past two decades and teach in my online program can be shared with many more people like you.

I know, I'm a good dude.

But why should you read on – and why should you also consider following my 10-week program in this book? My name is Marc McLean and I've been involved in weight training for the past 22 years.

I'm author of the 'Strength Training 101' book series, and those books have now reached over 20,000 readers around the world (and counting).

As you've already discovered, I also teach an online weight training and diet program, and I'm a fitness writer for world-leading health and wellness website Mind Body Green, aswell as The Good Men Project.

This 10-week program will help you lose fat, develop lean muscle, and get in great shape – if you put in the work. But everything I teach goes way beyond just the physical.

Your strength levels will go through the roof, as will your confidence in and out of the gym. You'll be more focused, driven, enthusiastic about your workouts, and most likely life in general.

These sound like bold assumptions from a guy you don't know, but I'm saying all of this with confidence because those are the positive benefits the men and women who go through my program experience.

Don't take my word for it, I'll be sharing the stories of six people I coached through the program from January-March 2020 later in this book.

Ordinary people just like you, who had exercise and diet struggles you can probably relate to aswell. So, I'm not going to be showing you muscled-up guys with six packs and super slim women covered in fake tan.

No, I'm talking about authentic stories that look past just the physical improvements. You'll hear them all talk about how the Be Your Own PT program completely changed their mindset, how they put in gym performances they thought weren't possible, and how the dedication and commitment to a healthy new lifestyle had a huge impact on other areas of their lives.

Another important benefit is the simplified dietary advice you'll learn in the upcoming chapters. In my experience, diet is the area where most people struggle.

Complicated meal plans, food restrictions, obsessive calorie counting...all of this takes the fun out of health and fitness. It's unsustainable – and it ultimately leads to people getting fed up and quitting.

You'll be pleased to know we do things completely differently around here. By the time you've finished reading this book you'll be equipped with a much simpler, effective approach to diet and nutrition that you can stick with in the long run.

I know because this is what I've been doing for many years. As for the people who have learned about my training methods and principles on diet, they often give me feedback about how they wished they'd discovered this way much sooner.

I want you to experience huge benefits from what I teach in this book too, and I'm going to make you a big promise right now...

You'll never have to rely on anyone else again when it comes to your fitness. As long as you implement everything in this book and put in the hard work in the gym, you can absolutely Be Your Own PT – and completely transform yourself physically and mentally.

Let's not hang around. The time is now, my friend.

Get through the upcoming chapters. Get inspired. Then get your ass into gear.

PART ONE
PREPARATION

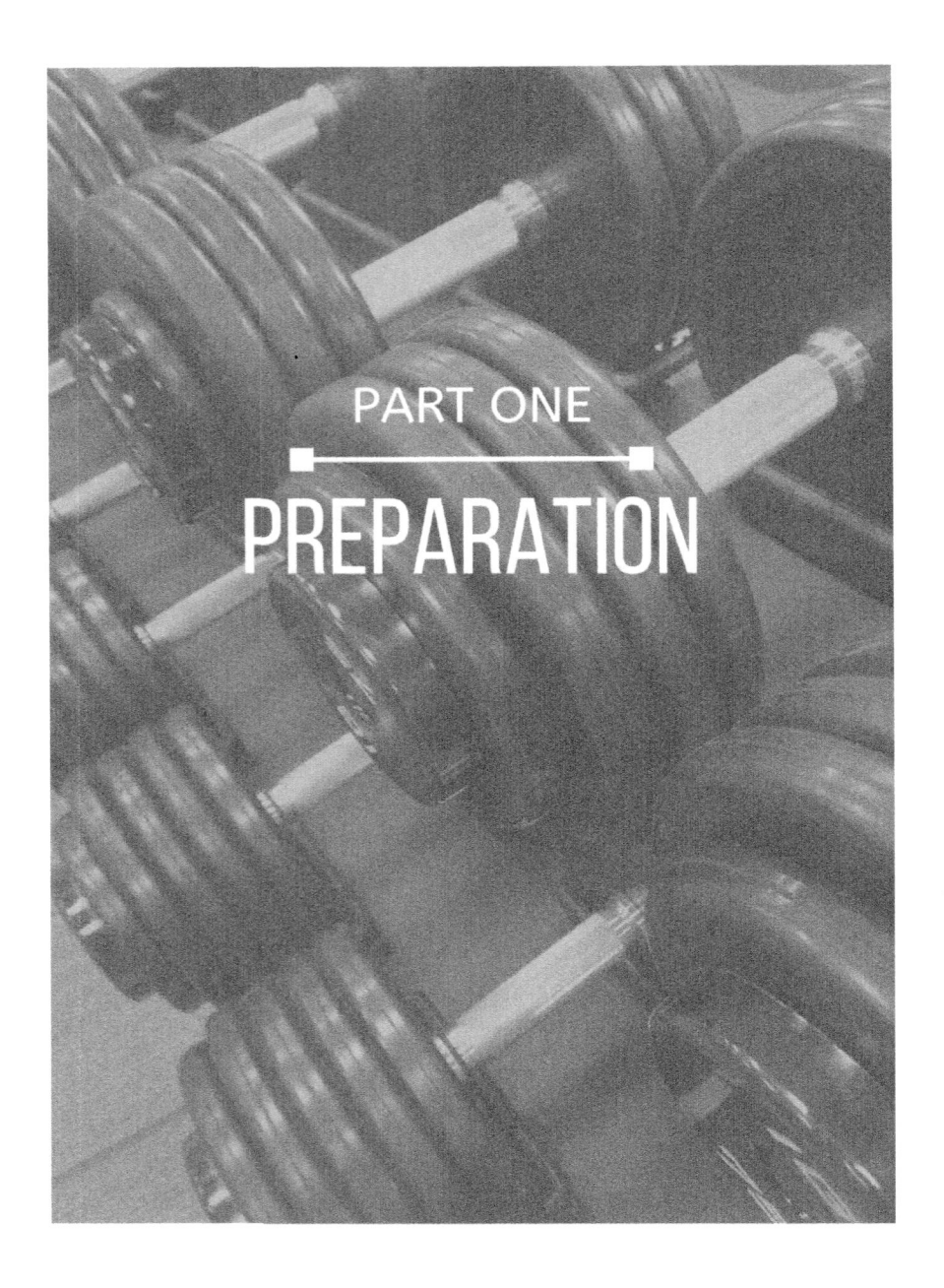

Chapter 1

PT vs Yourself

The guy huffed and puffed as he did another 50m lap on the gym carpet.

He trudged past me sweating with his legs tiring, ready to hop on the stationary exercise bike at the far end of the room next.

"C'mon, let's go," shouted the young personal trainer in her early 20s; at least half his age.

I was standing a few yards away completely confused. The guy looked sensible enough to me, but this scenario seemed bonkers.

It was January and he was being coached by a personal trainer to get back in shape. Roger that.

He was getting off his ass and doing something positive, rather than just laying about on the couch. Roger that too.

Here's where things didn't really make sense...

The guy was jogging up and down a stretch of carpet in the gym next to all the resistance machines.

Meanwhile, there were a row of treadmills down at the cardio section of the gym. There was also the perfect opportunity for jogging if he stepped back outside the door. It's free out there and so is the fresh air.

Thirdly, he was paying a personal trainer £20-£30 per hour for the privilege of jogging inside the gym...while she periodically shouted at him in a room full of 25 people.

And let's not forget the fact that jogging/running/hopping on an exercise bike are all ineffective ways of exercising if your January fitness goals are to burn fat and develop lean muscle.

Some personal trainers are tremendous and can be very helpful, especially if you're a complete beginner in the gym.

But wouldn't you prefer to take full charge of your own workouts? Wouldn't you like to take every bit of credit for the hard work you do in the gym? Wouldn't it be more satisfying if you mapped your own way to fitness greatness...without someone following you around in the gym telling you what to do next?

As someone with 22 years of gym experience and a fitness coach, I often get requests to do one-to-one PT sessions with people.

I always say no. Why? I don't do personal training. Walking round the gym joined at the hip with someone, pointing to exercise machines, and telling them what to do isn't my idea of fun.

But more importantly, it's disempowering for people like you. How can you expect to become stronger physically and mentally when you're taking the cue from someone else just to get through your workout routine?

I'm not knocking personal trainers. Some of them are my friends, and some of them are really good at what they do.

But while I don't know you, I do know that you're clever enough to learn weight training exercises on your own. If you're able-bodied and injury-free, I know you can make good progress in the gym just like the others. And I know for certain that you're way stronger than you think you are.

All you need is three main ingredients:

* The right training systems.

* A sensible way of eating that can be maintained.

* And a strong commitment to bettering yourself.

I can hand over the knowledge on a plate for the first two. The third is obviously up to you.

But there's another massssssive ingredient for you that can make all the difference between smashing your fitness goals – or falling flat on your face.

This ingredient is like the stock for your soup.

Like the water for your tea.

Like the...okay, it's getting a bit ridiculous now.

I'm talking about: **accountability**. Having accountability is crucial to your fitness success, and to be fair this is one of the main reasons most people hire a personal trainer. They simply want someone to answer to.

That's cool, but you can still have accountability in other ways. i.e. using a gym training diary with all your workouts mapped out, or finding a training partner and keeping each other on track.

This is why I do online group coaching instead of one-to-one PT sessions.

* I can pass on my knowledge so that you can go solo in the gym.

* You can get advice and support from a distance – and still be in charge of your own fitness.

* You are part of a community of other men and women chasing similar fitness goals...which is like accountability on steroids.

Pros and Cons of Personal Training

So, let's now quickly cover the pros and cons of personal training. Then you can be certain that you've picked up the right book and we can crack on with how you can Be Your Own PT.

Pros

* **Learning correct technique** – if you're a complete beginner, it might be useful for a few PT sessions to pick up the right form for exercises. Then again, you could watch a YouTube clip over and over again till you get it.

* **Avoiding injuries** – by mastering the technique of those exercises, and warming up properly under the guidance of a PT, it lessens your chances of injury.

***Accountability** – as discussed.

Cons

* **Cost** – where I live it can cost anywhere from £20-£40 for a 1 hour PT session, but if I lived in London or some parts of the US it would definitely be more.

* **Working to schedules** – you and your PT have got to work to a specific schedule. What if one of you are late? What if one of you are sick? What if someone cancels?

* **Disempowering yourself** – this is the biggest drawback in my opinion. You're an adult. You're able bodied. You can do this on your own.

* **Taking the easy path** – by relying on someone to lead the way in the gym, you're taking the easy path. Sure, you might not be that confident on your own at first...but that's where the growth comes.

When you do what you've not done before and step outside of your comfort zone, that's when you really start to make positive changes in your life.

Chapter 2

Weight Training // Intermittent Fasting // Accountability

This whole getting-in-great-shape thing is simple. There I said it.

"Easy for you to say, you're naturally slim..."

"But you've been doing this for years..."

"Blah, blah, blah."

When people say things like this, all I hear are excuses. The fact is, your gym workouts and a healthy approach to nutrition is simple – if you make it simple. I'm not saying it's easy, but it definitely can be straightforward.

Problem is, most people find complicated ways of going about things. It's no surprise because there's so much noise in the health and fitness world, with different experts saying so many different things that you don't know who to listen to.

My advice: do what has been *proven to work* for your particular fitness goals...what is *easiest to maintain*...and what you *enjoy* doing.

Since you picked up this book on weight training, I'm guessing that at a basic level you want to develop more lean muscle and keep your bodyfat levels low. An all-round, more athletic body. Correct?

* Weight training has long been proven to be highly-effective at developing muscle, and burning bodyfat at the same time.

* A weekly weight training routine like I recommend – just 3 x 1 hour sessions per week – definitely isn't hard to maintain. If you can't make that kind of time for yourself in your life, then you really don't have a life.

* Pushing yourself hard in the gym, becoming stronger week by week, and seeing steady progress can be hugely satisfying and enjoyable.

All 3 boxes ticked.

However, if you're doing the wrong exercises, training 5,6,7 days per week, and following one of these super high protein…or low carbs…or whatever the latest fad diet is, then life isn't going to be simple.

And the odds of you sticking with this sort of fitness program for long enough aren't very good…because it's difficult to maintain…and it's not very enjoyable.

Weight Training: Simplified

There was an American guy back in the 70s who ripped up the weight training rule book, and showed how it really should be done. He had a thick black moustache – proper 70s style – and a huge muscular body he'd developed for bodybuilding competitions.

While other bodybuilders at the time were training virtually seven days per week – and sometimes twice per day – the black moustache guy was lifting weights just every second day. Then further down the line he cut it down to just two days per week.

His name was Mike Mentzer, an all-natural athlete who won Mr Universe in 1978. Now while I'm definitely not into bodybuilding, I'm bringing up this story because Mike was a bit of a pioneer when it came to working out most efficiently and putting great emphasis on giving your body proper time to recover, repair and develop.

His approach was to give your all in the gym, lifting heavy and intensely to spark the hypertrophy (muscle growth) process, and then resting up right and eating properly to make the most of your hard gym efforts.

It makes sense, right? Lifting weights causes tiny tears on your muscle fibres, which is essentially tissue damage at a very small level. This leads to inflammation, which you feel as the soreness and stiffness the day after a good workout (and often the second day too).

Giving it 100% in your weight training workouts should naturally result in two-day soreness. Why hit the gym again the next day when it's very uncomfortable and your body is still in the process of bringing down the inflammation levels?

You might be keen to make more progress in less time, but this is actually counter-productive. Your body is still patching up those tiny muscle fibre tears, and by hitting the gym more than you need to you're interfering with that process.

Weight Training Frequency: Simplified

What's the answer? Lift weights every 48 hours. This means doing weight training just 3-4 days per week max; such as Mon, Wed, Fri or Tue, Thu, Sat, Mon.

There are countless weight training exercises out there that you can do to work virtually every muscle in the body. Ropes, band, cables, bars, handles have all been thrown into the mix along with dumbbells, barbells, kettlebells, and weighted plates of all shapes and sizes.

If you did all of those exercises in one session, you'd likely spend all day in the gym. But why work each muscle individually with one particular exercise when you can work 3,4,5 muscles at once with just one move?

That's what is possible when you introduce more compound exercises into your weight training workouts. That's been my approach from day one and, if you've read any of my other books in the 'Strength Training 101' series, you'll know I'm always banging on about compound exercises.

These are simply big multi-joint exercises that engage various muscle groups at once. i.e. the bench press works the chest, shoulders, triceps and forearms; upright row works the shoulders, trapezius, biceps and forearms.

Meanwhile, a popular exercise like the barbell curls simply work the biceps alone. Would you rather do 24 x exercises like the barbell curls to achieve an all-over body workout – or 6 or 7 compound moves to achieve the same goal in much less time?

Science has also shown that working various muscle groups at once in this synergistic way naturally produces more anabolic hormones, which is good news for your fat loss and muscle development goals.

Weight Training Exercises: Simplified

Therefore, simplifying the types of weight training exercises means including more compound exercises.

My top compound exercises are: bench press, bent over row, chin-ups, clean and press, deadlifts, dips, military press, pull-ups, squats.

I've created short demo videos to show you how to perform each of them on my Weight Training Is The Way YouTube channel: www.youtube.com/c/weighttrainingistheway

For easy access to these videos and ones I create in future, just hit the subscribe button on my YouTube channel.

In my Be Your Own PT 10-week program, we begin doing workouts that are comprised of compound exercises only. This is to build a strong foundation with the biggest and best exercises.

Weight Training Systems: Simplified

Of course, it would be mind-numbingly boring if all you did was rotate 10 exercises for 10 weeks straight. So we then gradually introduce very effective muscle isolation exercises week by week.

For example, in week 3 we add the dumbbell press (chest), lat pulldown (back/shoulders), triceps pushdown (triceps), and Arnie press (shoulders) into the mix.

By week 5, reverse flyes (rear shoulders), deltoid raises (front shoulders), lying bench curls (biceps), and pec deck (chest) all make an appearance in your workout plan too.

Having built that solid foundation with compound exercises that work the entire body, you will be well equipped by the time these muscle isolation moves are introduced.

These isolation exercises will help develop muscle definition in specific body parts. They'll also test you further in your workouts, and keep your gym sessions fresh and challenging. Exactly what we want!

For those very same reasons, I also switch training systems three times throughout the 10-week program. By 'systems' I mean a different approach to weight training in terms of your number of sets, rest periods between those sets, and amount of weight lifted.

For example, the first couple of weeks you'll simply do 3 x standard sets of each exercise, with 60 seconds rest in between each one.

However, for week 3 you'll switch to the 'The 3 Set Shocker'. This involves doing 2 standard sets, but immediately after the second set you'll decrease the weight by one third and then jump straight into doing your third set – with no more than 30 secs rest in between.

This 'shocks' the muscles – which have been used to a longer period of rest – into action and triggers more growth and development.

By week 6, you'll switch to the 'Drop Sets' training system and for weeks 8,9, and 10 you'll follow the 'Slow Burner' system.

I'll go into detail on each later in the book, but I'm just giving you a taster of what's to come – and underlining that this is a unique program I'm sure you're going to love.

We don't do run-of-the-mill, boring, repetitive workouts around here. After many years of experimentation, I've structured a 10-week program that's designed perfectly to:

* Keep you motivated and excited for every workout session

* Challenge you and bring the best out of you

* Avoid the dreaded training plateaus most people experience after a few weeks

* Ensure continuous, steady progress week by week by week

* Develop lean muscle, while lowering bodyfat levels at the same time

* Rack up a series of personal bests in the gym that give you immense satisfaction

* Take your strength to levels you didn't think were possible

Don't Just Take My Word For These Great Results...

That's a few bold claims I've just listed above. And Be Your Own PT is my program...so obviously I'm gonna say good things about it. But I don't expect you to just take my word for it.

Here are some of the comments that are posted underneath the video lessons as people have been progressing through the various weeks of the program.

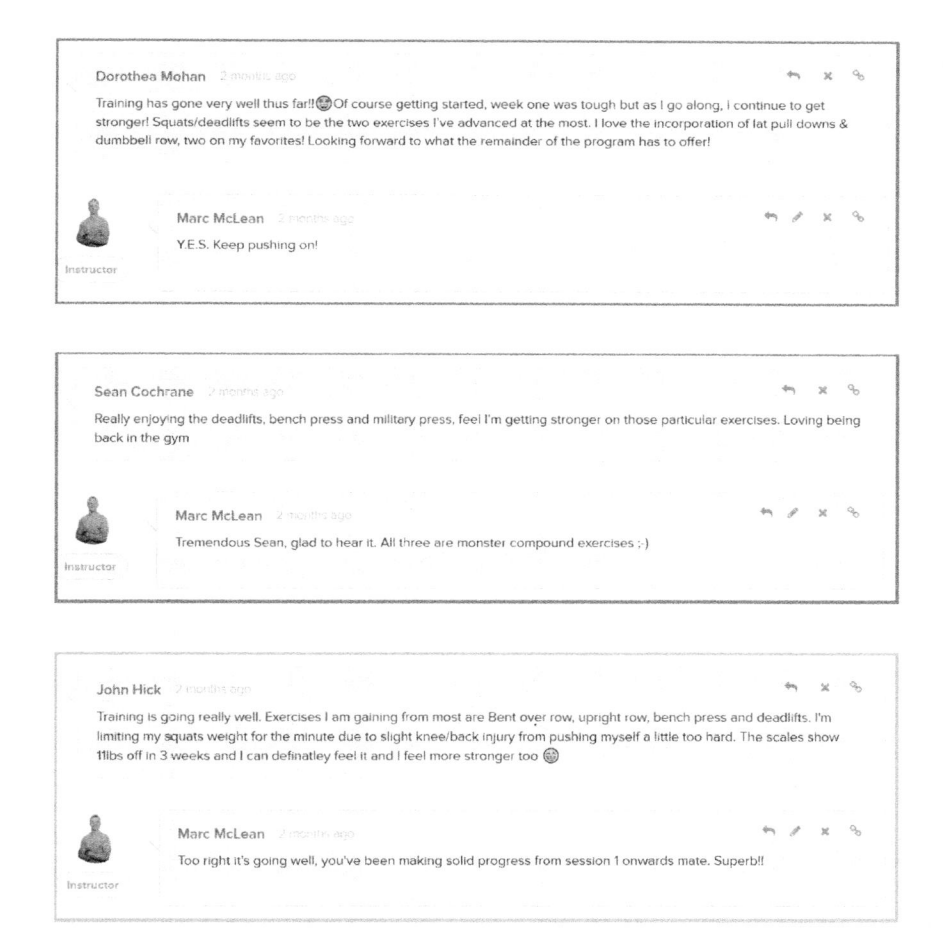

Dorothea Mohan 2 months ago

Training has gone very well thus far!! 😊 Of course getting started, week one was tough but as I go along, I continue to get stronger! Squats/deadlifts seem to be the two exercises I've advanced at the most. I love the incorporation of lat pull downs & dumbbell row, two on my favorites! Looking forward to what the remainder of the program has to offer!

Marc McLean 2 months ago
Y.E.S. Keep pushing on!
Instructor

Sean Cochrane 2 months ago

Really enjoying the deadlifts, bench press and military press, feel I'm getting stronger on those particular exercises. Loving being back in the gym

Marc McLean 2 months ago
Tremendous Sean, glad to hear it. All three are monster compound exercises ;-)
Instructor

John Hick 2 months ago

Training is going really well. Exercises I am gaining from most are Bent over row, upright row, bench press and deadlifts. I'm limiting my squats weight for the minute due to slight knee/back injury from pushing myself a little too hard. The scales show 11lbs off in 3 weeks and I can definatley feel it and I feel more stronger too 😊

Marc McLean 2 months ago
Too right it's going well, you've been making solid progress from session 1 onwards mate. Superb!!
Instructor

Intermittent Fasting: A Diet Revolution

Diet is the big problem. Of the many people I've helped with health and fitness – either by email, through my books, in person, or in group coaching – I'd estimate that around 80% of them struggle most with following a healthy diet.

What makes that even more problematic is that your nutrition is central to your results. You can work out like a warrior 365 days per year, but if you're eating fried chicken for breakfast and ice cream for dinner then your superhero gym efforts have been a complete waste of time.

This is the seventh book in my weight training series, and it's no surprise that my second book *Strength Training Nutrition 101: A Healthy Way Of Eating You Can Actually Maintain* is by far the best-selling title.

It's consistently been the most popular book every month for the past three years, and that reaffirms that diet is the sticking part for most men and women.

Here's the standard approach from 95% of health and fitness pros to help people looking to get in shape: cut your calories, cut out all your favourite treats, eat more of this, eat less of that.

The focus is all on *what* you are eating. This makes sense, and it does work…but for how long? There are two big problems here: *food restriction* and *limited willpower*.

Constantly counting calories, constantly struggling to resist foods you have regularly eaten, and constantly following a diet where there are restrictions are all naturally going to wear you down over time.

We only have limited willpower and it's also natural to have an inner resistance to restrictions placed upon us. This strain is heightened if you're following one of the latest trendy zero carb/high protein/whatever-you-call-them fad diets.

Therefore, it's only a matter of time before you crack - and then sprint to the nearest all-you-can-eat for £20 buffet. Then it's game over. Back to the start.

What makes my dietary approach in the Be Your Own PT program so successful is that you don't obsess over calories, you don't completely ban all your favourite foods, and you don't place all focus on what you eat.

You see, intermittent fasting is a big component of the program – and this puts emphasis on *when* you eat. By optimising your meal times – and eating sensibly, not restrictively – you can achieve amazing results *that you can maintain in the long run.*

How Intermittent Fasting Works

Your body's main source of energy is the glucose it derives from carbohydrates. Excess glucose is converted into glycogen and stored in the liver and muscle cells for a steady supply of energy later.

It's like a glycogen bank where your body takes deposits for energy throughout your day. But when that bank of glycogen runs out your body needs to look elsewhere for fuel.

Where does it turn to? Your fat stores! In a process called lipolysis, the body breaks down the fat stored in your white adipose tissue into free fatty acids in the bloodstream.

These released fatty acids are then used as your primary fuel source. For your glycogen bank to run out, it generally takes 12-14 hours. This occurs when you hit the fasted state and the amount of fatty acids in the bloodstream increases. Between 18 and 24 hours the number of fatty acids increases even further.

The ideal fasting period I recommend is 14-16 hours for five days per week. This is what I've been doing for six years and what I suggest in the Be Your Own PT program.

Don't be put off, thinking this will be difficult and that you'll go hungry each day. It's actually much easier than you'd expect.

Intermittent fasting can be easily implemented and successfully maintained simply by: **skipping breakfast.**

Forget all that garbage you've heard about breakfast being 'the most important meal of the day'. That might be true for five-year-old children who are still developing and need some nutrition before learning at school.

But I'm guessing your school days are well behind you now, and I'm pretty sure you won't pass out without having your bacon and eggs or bowl of cereal in the morning.

Instead, hang on in there until 12noon or 1pm, before you have your first meal of the day. If you do, you can potentially turn your body into a fat-burning machine.

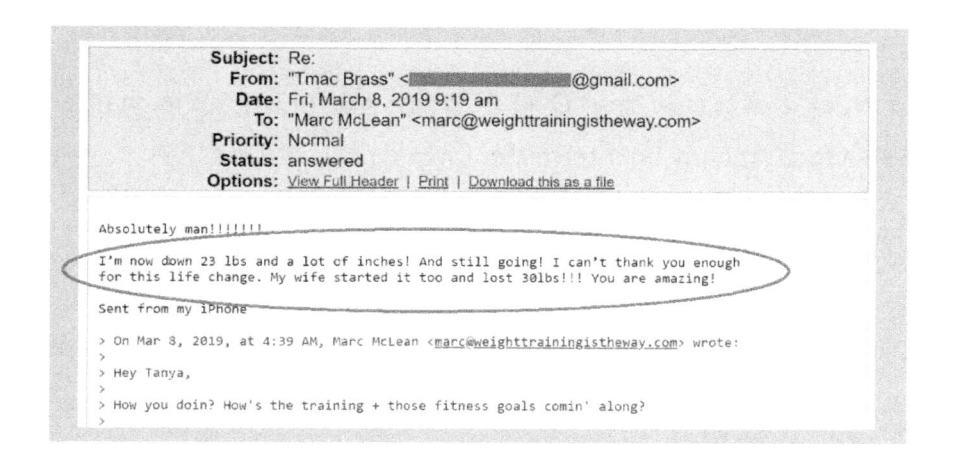

```
Subject: Re:
   From: "Tmac Brass" <             @gmail.com>
   Date: Fri, March 8, 2019 9:19 am
     To: "Marc McLean" <marc@weighttrainingistheway.com>
Priority: Normal
  Status: answered
 Options: View Full Header | Print | Download this as a file

Absolutely man!!!!!!!
I'm now down 23 lbs and a lot of inches! And still going! I can't thank you enough
for this life change. My wife started it too and lost 30lbs!!! You are amazing!

Sent from my iPhone

> On Mar 8, 2019, at 4:39 AM, Marc McLean <marc@weighttrainingistheway.com> wrote:
>
> Hey Tanya,
>
> How you doin? How's the training + those fitness goals comin' along?
>
```

This is an email I received from a woman in the US called Tanya McCann in March 2019. These were the results she got following intermittent fasting after learning about it in my book *Burn Fat Fast*.

I'm just showing you the picture above as proof that this is not all talk. Even big name stars, who are in ridiculously great shape, such as The Rock and Hugh Jackman, have been part of the intermittent fasting phenomenon.

I frequently get emails like the one above from people who have properly implemented my weight training and dietary advice. It feels great helping people to help themselves through what are essentially pretty simple tweaks to their lifestyle.

This is not dieting. Diets never last in the long run. Instead, intermittent fasting is a clever new way of eating that you can implement easily starting from today.

In Week 2 of the Be Your Own PT program (coming up in chapter 5) we focus mainly on intermittent fasting.

The Third Vital Component: Accountability

Okay, so we've covered a simplified, yet highly-effective approach to weight training, and a new way of eating that doesn't involve dieting and also focuses more on the timing of your meals.

There's also a third vital component in the Be Your Own PT program. One that's essential if you're serious about smashing your fitness goals. I'm talking about: accountability.

This of course means being held accountable to your fitness program, ensuring you do what you say you're going to do. It's all well and good being fired up in weeks one and two, but the action has got to continue for 10 weeks straight.

Willpower simply does not last that long. That's why you need gym workouts that are fresh and challenging. It's why you need a dietary approach that doesn't feel like a drag. And it's also why you need additional accountability tools to keep you locked in for the long haul.

"There's levels to this game," – this is a cool quote I've always loved from an American mixed martial arts fighter called Daniel Cormier. I'm a huge fan of the UFC and he was light heavyweight champion of the world at the time.

As Cormier was gearing up for a fight, he'd often say this quote to let his opponents know they were in trouble because they hadn't reached his level of wrestling, boxing, and dedication to training.

There are also levels to your fitness game and the standards you set for yourself. Let me walk you through those levels.

Baseline: saying you're going to train hard, improve your diet, and get in great shape.

Level 1: taking action and turning up at the gym.

Level 2: taking action and turning up at the gym – with a proper training plan in place.

Level 3: taking action with a training plan – but also having a training partner.

A fairly high number of people who set themselves fitness goals fail miserably. Research funded by the website bodybuilding.com several years ago indicated that around half of people in the US quit their fitness resolutions before February, and three quarters of the people fail to hit their overall targets.

There can be various reasons for fitness failure, including obvious factors such as following ineffective programs, poor diet, or quitting through injury.

But I'd be willing to bet my mum (and her dog) on it that the majority of the people involved in the fitness resolution quitters study I mentioned above were only at level 1 when it comes to accountability.

Just turning up at the gym and taking action isn't necessarily enough. That 'action' could mean a three-minute jog on the treadmill, wandering about the gym aimlessly because it's busy, picking up some dumbbells and doing half-hearted repetitions, before jumping on the ab roller and folding some belly flab while crunching your neck.

Unless you move up to level two – with a proper training plan in place too – your workouts may very well suck. In order to get the most out of your gym sessions, it's essential to have a training plan with order, structure, direction, and targets to beat.

You might convince yourself that you're working hard and putting in the required effort when you stroll into the gym unprepared, but you're not kidding me.

It's easy to map out your workouts for the week ahead in a pocket diary. While it might seem that executing this organised training plan may only give you a small boost, you'd be mistaken.

You're much less likely to skip exercises, or even a single set of those exercises, because your training diary is holding you accountable. You're also going to be on your A-game, working harder than usual, because you'll want to outdo your previous gym performances.

Best of all: you'll get a huge buzz each time you tick off exercises and mark down a new personal best in your training diary.

Doing all of this, over the course of a 10-week period, adds up to big results. Much bigger results than you'd get simply by showing up at the gym promising not to let yourself down.

The 3 Pillars Of The Be Your Own PT Program

So there you have it: weight training simplified, intermittent fasting, and accountability are the three pillars of the Be Your Own PT program. Without one or all of those pillars, everything falls apart.

We use these as a foundation for everything we do over the full 10-week program, and I'll be going into more detail in chapter 4 about what's covered in each of those weeks.

First, let's ponder over all the amazing benefits you can expect to experience when you get serious about your health and fitness.

Chapter 3

Various Fitness Goals, One Approach

I sat staring at my laptop in anticipation for what was about to drop into my inbox.

It was January 10th and it was game time for 10 people. Three Americans, three English people, three Scots...and another Scotsman living in Germany.

These were the people I'd signed up to my first ever New Year fitness resolution group coaching program. Twenty-one people had applied, but these 10 were the ones that convinced me they were committed to doing the necessary work to get results.

Don't know about you, but I don't like time wasters. It's a pain in the ass all-round when people don't back up their words with actions.

That's why I created an application process before kick-starting the 10-week group coaching program – so that I could weed out the half-hearted people.

Once I had my team of 10, it was time to get down to business. I was all-in for helping them become leaner, stronger, and to make

2020 the year that they smashed their New Year fitness resolutions.

But I needed to know exactly what they were aiming for. I needed honest answers about what their main stumbling blocks were when it came to exercising regularly and eating a healthy diet. I wanted to hear about the bad habits holding them back so we could overcome them.

The questionnaire I'd sent them that day would reveal all. And I was keen to read the answers to one question in particular. That's why I was sitting in front of my laptop impatiently waiting for their feedback to drop.

"Please list the top three things you want to achieve through this 10-week fitness program."

With five men, five women, and their ages ranging from 26 to 70, I wasn't too sure of the responses I'd receive to that question.

"More confidence. Muscle gain. Fat loss."

"A progressive increase in overall body strength. Gaining a better understanding of how to structure a week of training. Improve at exercises I've been doing for years but seeing little progress with."

"Build muscle. Become strong. Be able to do chin-ups."

"Fat loss, strength, consistency."

"Lower body fat percentage, change my lifestyle, get stronger and leaner."

"Lose weight and get to 180lbs or less. Get stronger. Feel stronger mentally and build confidence."

"Build muscle. Be fit. Be healthy."

"Build strength and overall tone. Tighten up my 'bat wings' (back of arms). I have 'chicken sticks' for legs…let's work on that."

"Weight loss. Tone and tighten body. Gain strength for pull-ups."

"Increase strength. Learn new weight training exercises. Fat loss."

There was a bit of everything in those responses. Fat loss, muscle gain, an exact target of weight loss, working on tightening particular body parts, becoming physically and mentally stronger, and learning how to be consistent with training.

With these people having different goals, and being a mix of different ages, abilities, shapes and sizes, you might be thinking that this makes it almost impossible for one single program to cater to everybody's needs.

I don't see it that way. In fact, there is a common theme that runs throughout everyone's fitness goals. A universal goal that these men and women share, and an ultimate fitness goal that you, me and everyone want…

An optimal ratio of muscle to bodyfat.

Let me explain. A middle-aged man with a beer belly and arms barely strong enough to hold a pint of beer obviously has a ratio that swings in favour of bodyfat.

A young woman who eats well and exercises regularly will have a better ratio of muscle to bodyfat than an unfit woman who likes too many takeaways and chocolate biscuits.

For our bodies to be healthy, strong, and perform optimally, we must all develop muscle strength and tone, and keep bodyfat levels in check, while supplying our bodies with good nutrition.

That's exactly what this 10-week weight training program delivers. At a core level, it hits the target for everyone.

And since there is a big emphasis on big compound exercises and working the entire body in each workout, the Be Your Own PT program is perfectly designed to help you achieve your other individual goals, whether that's women looking to tone their arms and legs, or men looking to lose the belly or become so strong that they can rattle out chin-ups like a pro.

The Be Your Own PT program will ultimately help you develop a leaner, stronger body with good overall composition.

And just for good measure, your strength levels will go through the roof, as will your confidence when you achieve what you never thought was possible in the gym.

By staying committed to the program and consistently showing up to each workout, each week, and overcoming excuses, you'll naturally develop your self-esteem and see a new-found positivity begin to infect other areas of your life.

You'll see what I mean when I share the remarkable stories of these men and women who completed the New Year program. You'll be inspired by what they achieved in that relatively short period running from the second week in January to mid-March.

The Path To Becoming Leaner & Stronger

The average man's body is made up of 18%-25% bodyfat, while women will carry 25%-32% bodyfat (mother nature gave women higher fat levels for reproduction and parenting).

It's once you go beyond these levels that you increase your risk of disease, your fitness levels drop, and you have less vitality.

Of course, the average bodyfat percentages will decrease further as you become stronger and more athletic through weight training, add more lean muscle, and increase your metabolism levels.

Let's be clear: while the ultimate goal is a better ratio of muscle to bodyfat, I never advocate neurotically measuring bodyfat levels with electrodes or any other fancy devices.

You won't need any fancy equipment, you'll know that ratio is improving by how firmer your body feels, how your overall body shape looks, and how your clothes fit you.

These are all clear indicators that you have a much better muscle:bodyfat ratio as a result of your dedication to lifting weights and eating cleaner.

With that one core ultimate goal in mind, I also split people who sign up to my Be Your Own PT program into two categories.

Category 1: People who need to focus more on weight loss.

Category 2: People who don't.

Either way, my training and nutrition system is largely the same overall, with straightforward tweaks for each of these categories.

Category 1 – people focusing more on weight loss

For people who are noticeably overweight, want to drop bodyfat levels, or perhaps have a particular weight target to reach, then a *daily calorie deficit* is necessary.

This is something that just about everyone in the fitness world can agree on. What many people disagree on is exactly how to do it (* hint: we don't do it the conventional way around here).

The average man should take in around 2500 calories per day to maintain their bodyweight, while for women that number is 2000 calories.

We all know that if you regularly take in more calories than you expend, you'll gain weight, while if you consistently use up more than you eat the weight will begin to fall off.

So, the best idea is to drastically cut the amount of food you eat to lose weight, right? Wrong.

You certainly don't have to go into starvation mode, and drastically cutting calories is never something I recommend.

I know of women who've been limiting themselves to just 1,000 calories per day in a desperate attempt to lose weight quickly. There are many guys barely eating much more because they mistakenly think that eating less food is the only way to fat loss.

The Be Your Own PT program offers up a few other fat loss solutions. In fact, it is designed in such a way that your body becomes a fat burning machine, while helping you become stronger and develop lean muscle at the same time.

Here's how this happens:

#1 Calories burned during your workouts – a good weight training workout can burn roughly 500 calories, sometimes more, on its own. People often don't appreciate how lifting weights fires up your metabolism.

#2 Your metabolism levels stay elevated much longer – research has shown that your metabolism stays heightened for 12-24 hours after a tough weights session, particularly when multi-joint compound exercises are in the mix. This means you continue to burn more calories on autopilot throughout the day.

#3 Intermittent fasting assists – as mentioned earlier, intermittent fasting forces your body to use up its fat stores for energy. You could literally be sitting at your desk in work mid-morning in a fasted state and your body will be breaking down fatty acids without any real effort from you.

#4 Intermittent fasting assists again – people on strict, calorie cutting diets limit themselves to a certain amount of calories per day and this has to be spread over breakfast, lunch, dinner and snacks.

However, with intermittent fasting you've already skipped breakfast, therefore you're already ahead of the game. This gives you more freedom to eat normally for the rest of the day without stressing that you're going to bust your calorie limit.

#5 Working out on an empty stomach – I recommend that people on my program do one or two gym workouts in the morning on an empty stomach where possible.

Training while fasted enhances the anabolic effects when you have your post-workout shake/meal an hour or so after finishing your workout.

The anabolic hormones develop muscle and strip away fat. Whatever you can do to help your body naturally produce more hormones such as growth hormone or testosterone will improve your health and fitness. (Women, don't worry. The testosterone won't turn you into a gorilla as your body is incapable of producing anywhere near the levels of men).

So to sum up, the five factors I've just listed help your body achieve a calorie deficit so that you can achieve fat loss – without having to drastically cut calories and follow a diet you hate.

Instead of cutting your calories by 1,000 or more per day, you could reduce them by just 300-400 and keep tabs on your daily intake for the first few weeks.

You could do this by doing a rough calculation in your head, or by using the handy MyFitnessPal app.

Either way, I don't think it's necessary or helpful to continually count calories for more than a few weeks. Some people become quite obsessed and it can drive you nuts.

After 2-3 weeks you'll have a fair idea of the amount of calories in common foods you eat and will be able to judge your daily intake without keeping track of every single thing that reaches your belly.

Category 2 – people who don't need to focus on weight loss

If you're someone who doesn't have weight to lose, and you simply want to develop more muscle definition, or improve your overall body shape, then you fall into the second category.

Same approach with weight training. Same approach with intermittent fasting. You simply have more freedom calorie wise. And if you're a naturally slim person like me, with a higher metabolism, then it'll be necessary to consciously eat more calories than the average person to develop muscle.

Personally, the easiest way to do this for me is by drinking a high calorie power shake every day and include more foods rich in healthy fats (which are also calorie dense), such as almonds, hummus, nut butters etc.

As for the high calorie power shakes, I include recipes for these in my previous books *Meal Prep* and also *The Meat Free Fitness Menu*.

It's Not About Six Pack Abs And The Perfect Body...

One guy was standing there looking like a mahogany statue of muscle with a newspaper in his hand.

Next to him was a photo of a woman in a bikini, with a pearly white smile, and also looking rather tense as she posed for the camera.

As I flipped to the next page, there were a bunch more men and women standing in various poses, showing off how they had transformed their bodies after a 16-week fitness program.

This was about 10 years ago, and I was considering giving the same program a bash because I wanted to try something new, and to give myself a target to really focus on.

But something just didn't feel right about it for me.

I quickly realised it was all those half-naked, flashy testimonial photos. Sure, these people had some great fitness achievements and they're to be applauded for their muscle gains and fat losses.

But the awkward looking, flexing poses? Holding newspapers to prove the date of their big body transformations? Covering themselves in fake tan and whitening their teeth?

It was all very contrived and off-putting. The thing I didn't like about it most was that it was putting all focus on one thing only: how these people looked.

Of course, you want to see clear positive changes in your body shape at the end of a lengthy fitness program. We all want more lean muscle and less fat, don't we?

But there are so many other huge benefits you can experience from lifting weights. There are also numerous other markers of success than just a semi-naked 'before' and 'after' photo. Whether you're caked in fake tan or holding a daily newspaper or not.

Strength training is not all about muscle, having a certain percentage of bodyfat, or six-pack abs. That's certainly not what I'm all about, or what this program is all about.

Success You Can Expect On The Be Your Own PT Program

Strength training can bring you a multitude of physical and mental benefits; some of which you probably didn't expect. I've experienced them myself over the past 22 years of lifting weights and witnessed the same with many men and women of all ages, shapes, sizes and abilities.

Looking beyond weight loss numbers, or the size of your legs or biceps, here are just some measures of success you can fully expect – if you put in the work.

* A rock-solid mindset.

* Improved mood and overall increase in positivity.

* Higher confidence levels.

* A boost in self-esteem and stronger self-image.

* More assertiveness in life outside of the gym.

* Improved health and wellbeing.

* A significant increase in strength levels.

* Conquering exercises you thought you'd never be able to do.

* Achieving numerous personal bests you never thought were possible.

Even experiencing just one or two of the above – particularly if you've been struggling with your health and fitness - can make a big difference to the quality of your life.

Experience them all and you're talking about a complete transformation that can positively influence other areas of your life, such as feeling more confident in close relationships or having the drive to go for a promotion in work.

It's been incredible for me to see people who follow this 10-week program really flourish. They become hooked on their weight training workouts, get excited about what's coming next, and take their confidence to the next level each week as a result of the clear progress they've made in the gym.

In part three of this book I'm certain you'll be able to relate to at least one of the case studies, and my hope is that it gives you a swift kick up the ass to get started on your own fitness and mindset transformation when you see what's really possible.

PART TWO
THE PROGRAMME

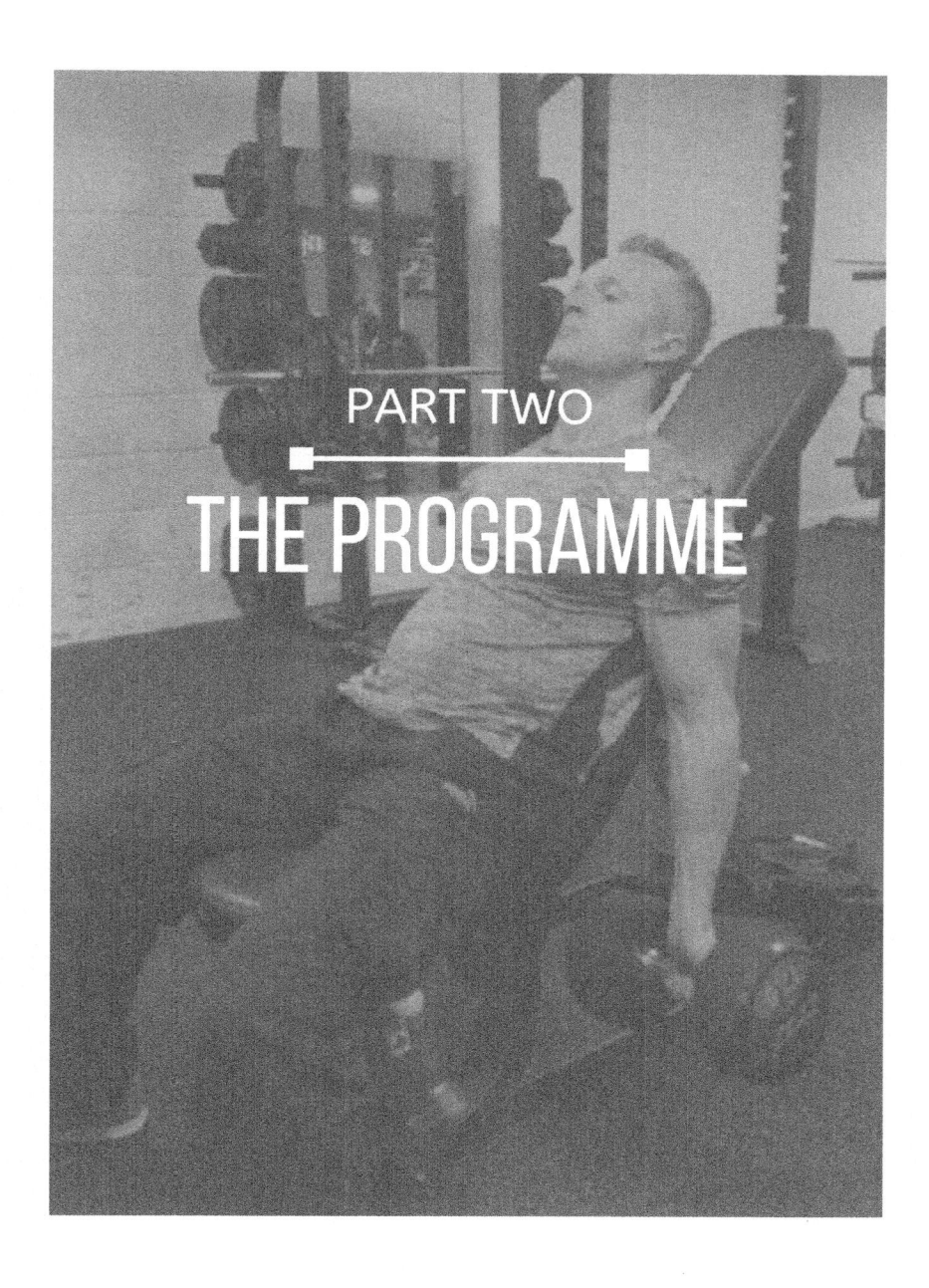

Chapter 4

Mastering The Compounds (Week 1)

The next 10 chapters will walk you through each week of the Be Your Own PT program.

Every week has a particular theme/area of focus, and there's a gradual progression with new concepts, fresh training systems implemented, new exercises introduced, nutritional advice, and a positive habit to maintain throughout that particular week.

The idea is that you're not bombarded with everything at once and feel overwhelmed. That would only lead to stress, struggle, and quitting by the time you reached week two or three.

This gradual weekly approach of implementing new weight training tactics, dietary steps, and positive habits makes it more enjoyable. It also makes it much more likely that you'll stick with the full 10-week program – and maintain these lifestyle changes long term.

The last thing I want is for you to trudge your way through the program for 10 weeks, and then revert back to old ways afterwards.

While this is a targeted program where you can mark a beginning and end date on your calendar, my wish is for all of this to become a new health and fitness lifestyle that keeps you strong, healthy and happy until you're 103 years old. Or thereabouts.

So, what's the theme/area of focus for Week 1? Mastering those compound exercises I'm always raving about. I'm crazy about compounds. You will be too once you realise how effective these multi-muscle movements are.

I'm talking about squats, deadlifts, bench press, chin-ups etc...those big, bold, old school exercises that work your body hard. Compounds should make up the majority of your gym workouts, anywhere from 60%-100% of your exercises for that day.

As compound exercises are a central part of your training, we begin week 1 by introducing the best compound moves and learning how to master them.

After we look closely at the theme for each week, the following four areas are covered:

#1 Your training plan of 3 x gym workouts for the week ahead, including exercises, training system, number of sets, rest period etc.

#2 Nutritional advice – this doesn't begin until week two (as it's so important you focus solely on mastering the compounds for now).

#3 Accountability tactics – small but important steps you can take each week to help stay on track.

#4 Weekly positive habit – this will be something fairly simple that you implement, but you must follow this habit religiously for the week.

We then introduce a new positive habit the following week, same again the following week, and we begin stacking these positive habits up on top of one another.

By the end of the full 10-week program those small habits have added up to big results.

Starting Strong With The 10 Compounds

By working various muscle groups at once, compound exercises deliver an efficient all-over body workout. Studies have also shown that doing compound exercises with increasingly heavy weight increase the production of anabolic hormones, which results in more muscle and less fat.

The following 10 brilliant compound exercises (in no particular order) are included in this program:

* Squats.

* Deadlifts.

* Bench press.

* Military press.

* Bent over row.

* Upright row.

* Chin-ups (done with assistance until you become stronger).

* Pull-ups (also done with assistance until you develop upper body strength).

* Dips (also done with assistance at the beginning).

* Clean and press.

You'll be focusing primarily on these in your 3 workouts in week 1, and again the following week.

But don't worry, we'll be mixing up the order of the exercises to keep things fresh and challenging, and in upcoming weeks we'll also be introducing plenty of muscle isolation exercises…and switching up training systems several times too.

Week 1 Workouts

Coming up I'll set out your three weight training workouts for the week ahead. I suggest you buy a pocket-book or use the notes app on your mobile phone to create a gym training diary. Then jot down the upcoming three workout plans in the same format as I'm about to lay out.

* **Training system** – this will change every 2-3 weeks.

* **Exercise** – simply the name of each exercise.

* **Sets** – number of sets you should do of each exercise, and this will be 3 for the duration of the program.

* **Reps** – repetitions in each of those sets, and you should always aim for between 6 and 9. If you can do 9 or more comfortably, then increase the weight for your next set.

If you struggle to reach six, then decrease the weight a little. (Remember, proper exercise technique should always be a priority...never sacrifice good technique just to lift more weight).

* **Rest** – this refers to the rest period in between each set of your exercises. The standard is 60 secs, but this will fluctuate depending on which training system you're following on a particular week.

You'll note that I have leave the 'weight' and 'notes' fields blank. This is for you to fill in as you go along in the gym. It's up to you to experiment with different weight levels at the beginning to find the sweet spot for what you can manage at first.

Start off lighter at first in Week 1, focusing primarily on mastering the correct form of the compound exercises. Thereafter aim for 6-9 reps, using this range as a guide for the ideal weight you should be lifting.

By taking this approach you'll also increase your strength rapidly through progressively overloading the muscles with more weight, week-by-week.

* Importantly, you can then also set yourself targets of more reps and lifting more weight, and start marking down personal bests in your training diary.

I use the notes section to mark 'PB' for personal best whenever I've performed better on a particular exercise compared to previous workouts. I highly recommend doing the same as it'll take your training and results to the next level.

Important Safety Steps Before Beginning Your Workouts

#1 Always warm up well. Warm up for at least 4-5 mins before beginning your gym workout. Do a light jog on the treadmill for 2-3 mins to get the blood flowing, and then do some basic stretches for your legs and upper body.

It's also recommended that you do some really light weight repetitions of exercises you plan on doing in that workout. (i.e. a set of 10 upright row using the bar only, with no weights).

#2 Always put safety first. Remember to put safety collars on the bar to lock weights in place. Use safety bars at the squat rack when doing squats. Have someone act as 'spotter' – watching over and supporting you – as you do heavier lifts of the bench press.

#3 Always maintain good technique. Never compromise good form in any exercise in order to lift heavier weights. This will increase your chances of injury and will limit your overall progress.

#4 Watch the video demos. Because I want to ensure you learn proper technique and minimise risk of injuries, I've created short video clips of every exercise included in the program and made them available to you for free.

You can watch them here:

http://www.youtube.com/c/WeightTrainingIsTheWay

Remember to watch those clips before beginning any exercise you're unsure of. These will guide you and flag up common mistakes to avoid.

I've also included an Exercises Guide Index with pictures of me performing every exercise. You can find this at the end of the book.

Gym Workouts

Week 1, Workout 1

TRAINING SYSTEM – Three Sets Heavy

EXERCISE	SETS	REPS	REST	WEIGHT	NOTE
Squats	3	6-9	60 secs		
Deadlifts	3	6-9	60 secs		
Bench press	3	6-9	60 secs		
Assisted chin-ups	3	6-9	60 secs		
Military press	3	6-9	60 secs		
Upright row	3	6-9	60 secs		
Bent over row	3	6-9	60 secs		
Clean & press	3	6-9	60 secs		

Week 1, Workout 2

TRAINING SYSTEM – Three Sets Heavy

EXERCISE	SETS	REPS	REST	WEIGHT	NOTE
Bench press	3	6-9	60 secs		
Assisted dips	3	6-9	60 secs		
Bent over row	3	6-9	60 secs		
Upright row	3	6-9	60 secs		
Clean & press	3	6-9	60 secs		
Assisted chin-ups	3	6-9	60 secs		
Military press	3	6-9	60 secs		

Week 1, Workout 3

TRAINING SYSTEM – Three Sets Heavy

EXERCISE	SETS	REPS	REST	WEIGHT	NOTE
Squats	3	6-9	60 secs		
Deadlifts	3	6-9	60 secs		
Bench press	3	6-9	60 secs		
Assisted chin-ups	3	6-9	60 secs		
Military press	3	6-9	60 secs		
Upright row	3	6-9	60 secs		

| Bent over row | 3 | 6-9 | 60 secs | | |
| Barbell curls | 3 | 6-9 | 60 secs | | |

Nutrition

This week I postpone nutritional advice and I do this for two reasons. Firstly, I want you to focus solely on mastering the compound exercises in the gym.

Secondly, next week's entire theme will be based on nutrition. We'll be covering...

* The amazing benefits of intermittent fasting, and how you can easily implement it into your life to burn fat easily while developing muscle.

* Calorie intake.

* And solid nutritional principles that'll you find manageable and will help you sculpt a leaner, stronger body.

Accountability

There are several accountability steps you can take to keep you focused and on track...

* Make sure you fill in your gym training diary completely as you go along in the gym. Mark down the weights you lift, and the number of repetitions in each set in your diary's notes section. This will give you targets to beat and help you make steady progress.

* Complete a weekly review in your gym diary at the end of the week. Give yourself weekly scores out of 10 for your training, your diet, and your quality of sleep. Then write down one thing that worked really well, one thing you can improve upon, and also jot down how many personal bests you achieved in total for the week.

Doing this will help you assess how the week has gone, enjoy the wins, and identify anything you can improve upon for next week.

Your Weekly Positive Habit

Your positive habit for this week: make sure you complete all 3 gym workouts. No skipping any of them and fill in your diary as you go along in the gym.

Action Step To Take Right Now

Either order a pocket notebook if you don't already have one, or set up a digital gym training diary on your mobile phone notes app.

Once you have that diary, jot down your three workouts for the week ahead so that you're well prepared for a solid, laser-focused week of weight training.

Chapter 5

Intermittent Fasting (Week 2)

If you've never heard of intermittent fasting until you picked up this book and you're feeling quite excited, then you should be.

If you're someone who has struggled with dieting and want to try a new healthy approach, intermittent fasting could be perfect for you. I'm not promising miracle fat loss because I don't know all of your circumstances, but implementing this way of eating can be extremely effective if done properly alongside a good fitness regime.

And if you're just looking to stay lean, develop muscle definition, and improve your overall health, then intermittent fasting is just the job for you too.

Here's the game plan for Week 2. First we're going to look at the best way to implement intermittent fasting with this program. We'll also cover the amazing benefits of this way of eating.

Then we'll dive into my *Six Golden Rules of Clean Eating*. Forget boring diet plans, or counting every macronutrient, because combining solid nutritional principles with intermittent fasting will get you great results.

Then we'll quickly look at calories and figuring out your daily intake (but keeping it simple without any geeky or scientific crap).

Finally, just like every other week of the program, we'll lay out your gym workouts, nutritional advice, and accountability plan for the week ahead. And of course we'll wrap up with your positive habit for the week and an action step to take right away.

Implement Intermittent Fasting Easily By Skipping Breakfast

The ideal fasting period for burning fat effectively without eating into your muscle is around 14-16 hours. I'm personally around the 16-hour mark on my fasting days, but women should be closer to 14 hours and generally not exceed 16 hours. I'll explain why soon.

You've already been fasting, technically, during your sleep so by skipping breakfast and extending that fasted period further you can hit that 16-hour target.

For example, if you stop eating at 8pm, skip breakfast the next day, and don't have your first meal of the day until 12 noon, then that's 16 hours without food.

But this is totally flexible too. Say you were working late and didn't finish your dinner till 9pm. Skip breakfast again the next day, and simply hold off until 1pm before you have your lunch. Again, that's 16 hours. Bingo!

Of course, a fast bans food. Unfortunately that also means no coffee or tea with sugar, sweeteners or milk.

Black coffee, black tea, green tea, or water only.

It's not as hard as it sounds. Your stomach might grumble after the first few days without breakfast, but your body quickly adapts.

But one important point: only do intermittent fasting Monday-Friday, and eat as normal at weekends, because studies have shown that fasting loses its effectiveness when done continually.

Fasting: The Do's And Don'ts

Intermittent fasting is not dangerous or unhealthy; quite the opposite. Remember, this is the way our ancestors ate. Back in the hunter-gatherer days, humans would typically be out for long chunks of the day hunting and foraging.

Feasting wouldn't occur until the evening, which meant that intermittent fasting was a natural part of their lifestyle.

These days there are fast food places in every town and our supermarkets are filled with snacks and junk food that people can graze on all day.

It's no surprise that obesity is at epidemic levels in the US, and type II diabetes, heart disease etc are rampant in many Western countries.

Anyway, back to intermittent fasting. There are some important things to do and things to avoid in order to get the most out of this approach to eating.

DO...

* Be flexible with it – which means your eating window doesn't have to be set in stone each day. (You could fast between 8pm and 12noon one day, and then 9.30pm and 12.30pn the next. As long as there is a **14-16 hour** fasting period, you're hitting the sweet spot).

* Stick with it – if your stomach grumbles and you find it a struggle at first, don't worry because the body soon gets used to this way of eating after a few days.

DON'T...

* Fast 7 days per week – this is because the body will adapt and it'll become less effective. I recommend fasting Monday-Friday only, and then having breakfast as normal at weekends.

* Fast beyond 16 hours **women** – some research has suggested that fasting excessively along with calorie restriction can cause

hormone imbalances and affect menstrual cycles. So it's not recommended to exceed 16 hours, 14-15 hours is better.

* Have sugar or milk in your tea/coffee during fasting periods — while these drinks are not technically food, this will spike your blood sugar levels and mess up your fast. Have black tea/coffee or, even better, green tea instead.

There are also several key health benefits of intermittent fasting, which I cover in more detail in my book Fitness Hacking, but I'll simply list a few of them here. If you decide you want to learn more about any of them, then Google is your friend my friend.

* **Protects against brain disorders.**

* **Helps prevent killer diseases including heart disease, cancer, and obesity.**

* **Increases growth hormone levels.**

* **Keeps your heart healthy.**

* **Reduces inflammation in the body.**

* **Improves sports performance.**

***Aids detoxification.**

Plenty of reasons to skip breakfast and feel the benefits of intermittent fasting. But remember, that 14-16 hours is an ideal fasting period and to do it for just five days per week. Continuously fasting for longer periods than this may actually slow down your metabolism.

Six Golden Rules Of Clean Eating

#1 Cut out sugar as much as possible. Put plainly excess sugar is literally converted to bodyfat. Natural sugars from fresh fruit – yes, the sugars in sweets, chocolate and junk food...reduce those as much as you can.

#2 Eat more fruit and vegetables. These provide the vitamins, minerals, and tools your body needs maintain good health and wellness. Try to include fruit or vegetables with every meal you have, these should be your main sources of carbohydrates rather than processed foods.

#3 Cook fresh as much as you can. When you cook using fresh ingredients you know exactly what's going into your meals. There'll be no dodgy additives, preservatives, e-numbers etc, and you can opt for more healthy whole foods, along with natural spices to give your food some great flavor.

#4 Drink plenty of water. It's a good idea to invest in a 1 litre water bottle because women should be drinking 2 – 2.5 litres of water each day, while men should take in around 2.5 – 3 litres.

Sounds like a lot, but it's manageable if you fill up that water bottle a couple of times per day and take regular sips.

#5 Beware of the long ingredients list. Most pre-packaged foods in supermarkets have a huge list of ingredients and this is something to be wary of as some of these can be unhealthy colourings and additives like I mentioned above.

If there are too many weird long names included in the ingredients list, such as azodicarbonamide or sodium carboxymethyl cellulose, then best steering clear. Additives like these can disrupt your body's hormones and are toxic in big amounts.

#6 Ditch your microwave. This might sounds like a drastic move, but microwaves are a form of electromagnetic radiation – and these literally zap the goodness out of your food. A healthy meal that goes in the microwave comes out unhealthier.

Gently re-heating previously cooked meals can usually be done in a pot on the cooker instead.

Figuring Out Your Rough Calorie Intake

Calories is a contentious issue because many fitness professionals, diet plans, and people following those plans put a huge focus on counting calories.

Everyone knows that if you eat too many calories consistently you'll gain weight, and if you don't eat enough you'll lose weight.

That's why most fad diets are based around calorie counting, and food restrictions. But most diets fail in the long run - and there's far more to getting in great shape than just calories in and calories out.

Like I mentioned earlier, intermittent fasting will have you burning fat on autopilot, and weight training will increase your metabolism levels and burn more calories overall.

And for every pound of muscle you gain, your body burns around 35-50 calories just to maintain it.

So that's why in my program we never obsess over counting every calorie, we don't count protein, carbs and fats down to the gram in every meal, and we never restrict any foods completely.

Where's the fun in doing things like that? And who wants to live like that? It'll only leave you pissed off…and you'll end up going on junk food benders in Pizza Hut.

Instead, we're going to simplify your nutrition each week – so that you can actually maintain it in the long run. That will simply involve:

* Eating clean Monday-Friday and relaxing your diet at the weekends (without going too nuts).

* Following those Six Golden Rules Of Clean Eating we covered earlier.

* Doing intermittent fasting (aka skipping breakfast) Monday-Friday, and just eating breakfast normally again at weekends.

It's as simple as that. As you might expect, I'd recommend buying a good protein powder to drink 1 hour after you finish your workouts. But I'm going to go into more detail on supplements in the next chapter.

So, once again, it's not necessary to count calories obsessively. Instead, it's a smart move to know *roughly* how many calories your body requires each day and get to know *roughly* what's in common foods you eat. Then you can always stay within a healthy range.

None of this is an exact science, and the calorie counting brigade who try to make it so only end up making life more difficult in my opinion. Here's a simple calculation for figuring out roughly how many calories an average active person requires.

Weight loss: *Bodyweight in lbs x 12 = number of calories*

Weight gain: *Bodyweight in lbs x 17 = number of calories*

Maintenance: *Bodyweight in lbs x 15 = number of calories*

Therefore, the sums for 160lb guy aiming to gain weight and size while building muscle would shoot for around 2,700-2,800 calories (160 x 17 = 2,720).

Or a 170lb woman looking to lose fat would aim for 2,000 calories per day or less (170 x 12 = 2,040).

But if you're looking for a way for everything to be worked out for you, along with a more detailed look at the nutrition in the foods you're eating each day, then I'd recommend downloading the MyFitnessPal app.

It's really easy to use – and it's free. It's good for someone starting out to get to grips with the general numbers of calories and nutrients in their foods, but it's not essential and further down the line when you're more clued-up about what's in the common foods you're eating you won't need it anyway.

Gym Workouts

Sticking with compound exercises once again this week in order to master them. However, to turn things up a notch we're adding in a 'finisher' exercise at the end of your workouts.

This involves doing 5 sets of a particular exercise for 9 repetitions...with half the usual weight you would lift. This sounds fairly easy, but you're only allowed 10 secs rest in between each of those 5 sets.

That's why it's called the 'finisher': it really fatigues the muscles and you'll definitely feel finished once it's done! There's also a new exercise appearing in workout 3 this week.

Remember to copy these workout plans and jot them down in your training diary. Never step into the gym without a proper plan of action.

Week 2, Workout 1

TRAINING SYSTEM – Three Sets Heavy

EXERCISE	SETS	REPS	REST	WEIGHT	NOTE
Squats	3	6-9	60 secs		
Deadlifts	3	6-9	60 secs		
Bench press	3	6-9	60 secs		
Assisted chin-ups	3	6-9	60 secs		
Military press	3	6-9	60 secs		
Upright row	3	6-9	60 secs		
Bent over row	3	6-9	60 secs		
Clean & press	3	6-9	60 secs		
FINISHER: Light squats	5	9	**10 secs** (half weight, only 10 secs rest)		

Week 2, Workout 2

TRAINING SYSTEM – Three Sets Heavy

EXERCISE	SETS	REPS	REST	WEIGHT	NOTE
Bench press	3	6-9	60 secs		
Assisted dips	3	6-9	60 secs		
Bent over row	3	6-9	60 secs		
Clean & press	3	6-9	60 secs		
Assisted chin-ups	3	6-9	60 secs		
Upright row	3	6-9	60 secs		
Barbell curls	3	6-9	60 secs		
FINISHER: Light squats	5	9	**10 secs** (half weight, only 10 secs rest)		

Week 2, Workout 3

TRAINING SYSTEM – Three Sets Heavy

EXERCISE	SETS	REPS	REST	WEIGHT	NOTE
Deadlifts	3	6-9	60 secs		
Squats	3	6-9	60 secs		
Upright row	3	6-9	60 secs		
Military press	3	6-9	60 secs		
Bent over row	3	6-9	60 secs		

Assisted chin-ups	3	6-9	60 secs		
Cable row	3	6-9	60 secs		
FINISHER: Upright row	5	9	**10 secs** (half weight, only 10 secs rest)		

* Hit the gym 3 times this week and follow along the workouts in your training diary.

* Train 1 day on, 1 day off (such as Mon, Wed, Fri).

* Don't be skipping any workouts!

Nutrition

* Do intermittent fasting Mon-Fri, aiming for a fast of 14-16 hours. Remember, this is easily done by skipping breakfast.

* Relax your diet a little at the weekend. Have a takeaway meal if you like, and the odd treat after working hard in the gym. Remember not to do intermittent fasting at the weekend too.

* Follow the golden rules of clean eating (cut out sugar as much as you can, eat more vegetables and fruit, cook fresh as much as possible, drink enough water each day, beware of the long ingredients list and dodgy additives in foods, and don't microwave your food).

Accountability

* Make sure you fill in your gym training diary completely as you go along in the gym. Mark down the weights you lift and the number of repetitions in each set in your diary's notes section. This will give you targets to beat and help you make steady progress.

* Complete the weekly review in your gym diary at the end of the week. This will help you assess how the week has gone, enjoy the wins, and identify anything you can improve upon next week.

Positive Habit

* Make sure you do intermittent fasting every day Mon-Fri.

Action Step

* Work out your rough daily calorie intake. Either grab a notepad and do the calculation I explained earlier in this chapter, or download the MyFitnessPal app and use its settings that works out calories for you.

Chapter 6

The Three Set Shocker (Week 3)

Doing the same old workouts are not only boring, they limit your progress in the gym. That's why we always switch things up around here, and the big change this week is the introduction of the 'The Three Set Shocker' training system.

By system, I mean the particular approach you'll be taking in terms of your exercise sets, the weight lifted, and rest period after each set.

For the previous two weeks, it was a straightforward 3 sets and 60 secs rest after each one of them. Here's how The Three Set Shocker is different:

* You do your first two sets as normal with a heavy weight you can manage for 6-9 reps, with 60 secs rest in between those two sets.

* However, after your second set, reduce the overall weight of the exercise by around one third.

* Then jump straight into your third set of the exercise after only 20-30 secs rest, instead of 60 secs.

The idea with this is that the lack of rest shocks the body as this is not what it's been used to for the previous two weeks, and by testing the muscles this way you'll be encouraging muscle and strength development.

Gym Workouts

Roughly the same amount of exercises every week. Still 3 sets of each exercise. Still 6-9 reps, and a finisher exercise thrown in at the end for good measure.

The only difference is the change of training system – and five new muscle isolation exercises introduced to keep things fresh and challenging.

Those new exercises are: dumbbell flyes (chest); dumbbell press (chest); lat pulldown (back); Arnie press (shoulders); and triceps pushdown (triceps, you might've guessed).

Remember you can watch video demonstrations on how to perform every exercise at:
http://www.youtube.com/c/WeightTrainingIsTheWay

And, as always, write these workout plans down in your gym training diary in advance of working out.

Week 3, Workout 1

TRAINING SYSTEM – The Three Set Shocker

EXERCISE	SETS	REPS	REST	WEIGHT	NOTE
Bench press	3	6-9	60 secs		
Dumbbell flyes	3	6-9	60 secs		
Clean & press	3	6-9	60 secs		
Upright row	3	6-9	60 secs		
Assisted chin-ups	3	6-9	60 secs		
Barbell curls	3	6-9	60 secs		
Lat pulldown	3	6-9	60 secs		
<u>FINISHER:</u> Light dumbbell flyes	5	9	10 secs (half weight, only 10 secs rest)		

Week 3, Workout 2

TRAINING SYSTEM – The Three Set Shocker

EXERCISE	SETS	REPS	REST	WEIGHT	NOTE
Squats	3	6-9	60 secs		
Deadlifts	3	6-9	60 secs		
Cable row	3	6-9	60 secs		
Arnie press	3	6-9	60 secs		
Bent over row	3	6-9	60 secs		

Upright row	3	6-9	60 secs		
FINISHER: Light cable row	5	9	**10 secs** (half weight, only 10 secs rest)		

Week 3, Workout 3

TRAINING SYSTEM – The Three Set Shocker

EXERCISE	SETS	REPS	REST	WEIGHT	NOTE
Dumbbell press	3	6-9	60 secs		
Dumbbell flyes	3	6-9	60 secs		
Assisted chin-ups	3	6-9	60 secs		
Clean & press	3	6-9	60 secs		
Upright row	3	6-9	60 secs		
Assisted dips	3	6-9	60 secs		
Triceps pushdown	3	6-9	60 secs		
FINISHER: Light dumbbell press	5	9	**10 secs** (half weight, only 10 secs rest)		

* Hit the gym 3 times this week and follow along the workouts in your training diary.

* Train 1 day on, 1 day off (such as Mon, Wed, Fri).

* Don't be skipping any workouts!

NOTE: The following advice on nutrition and accountability will be the same every week for the remainder of the program, and so it might seem repetitive that the same information is always included at the bottom of each chapter.

However, I'm doing this intentionally as a reminder of the importance of these steps every week, and also because repetition of the right actions leads to best results.

Meanwhile, the positive habit action step at the very end of each chapter will be different each week, so please pay close attention.

Nutrition

* Do intermittent fasting Mon-Fri, aiming for a fast of 14-16 hours. Remember, this is easily done by skipping breakfast.

* Relax your diet a little at the weekend. Have a takeaway meal if you like, and the odd treat after working hard in the gym. Remember not to do intermittent fasting at the weekend too.

* Follow the golden rules of clean eating (cut out sugar as much as you can, eat more vegetables and fruit, cook fresh as much as possible, drink enough water each day, beware of the long ingredients list and dodgy additives in foods, and don't microwave your food).

Accountability

* Fill in your gym training diary completely as you go along in the gym. Mark down the weights you lift and the number of repetitions you managed in each set in your diary's notes section. This will give you targets to beat next time around and ensure solid progress.

* Complete a weekly review in your gym diary at the end of the week. Give yourself weekly scores out of 10 for your training, your diet, and your quality of sleep. Then write down one thing that worked really well, one thing you can improve upon, and also jot down how many personal bests you achieved in total for the week.

Doing this will help you assess how the week has gone, enjoy the wins, and identify anything you can improve upon for next week.

Positive Habit

* Buy a 1 litre water bottle and ensure you drink enough water each day this week, whether that's 2 – 2.5 litres for women, or 2.5 – 3 litres for men.

Chapter 7

Time For Some Personal Bests (Week 4)

If you're going to train in the gym, you may as well train like a warrior. Forget all this messin' about, mediocre stuff…it's time to take things to the next level.

I'm talking about really pushing yourself hard to achieve some personal bests. Fitness, sports, exercise…none of it would be much fun without competition.

Don't worry about what how many reps the person next to you is doing, or how much weight the guy standing at the squat rack is lifting. No, forget everyone else. I want you to compete with *yourself* in the gym.

Did 60kg on barbell squats last week? Let's try to achieve 9 good reps, and increase the weight to 65kg.

Managed a total of 17 assisted chin-ups over three sets in your last workout? Push yourself hard to try and do 1 or 2 more in your gym sessions this week.

This week I want you to aim for 3 personal bests in each workout.

You can now see why I stress the importance of using a gym training diary. It helps you keep track of your weights, number of reps, and setting targets like these. Working out this way fires you up in the gym – and you'll leave the place buzzing after you see what you're really capable of.

By this point in Week 4, if you've been working hard and following my advice, I have zero doubt you'll be much stronger now. This is prime time for pushing yourself and going beyond your previously self-imposed limits.

Mark down 'PB' in the notes section of your gym training diary each time you are able to increase the weight after a set of 9 reps on any exercise. For the bodyweight exercises (assisted chin-ups and dips), record the total amount of reps from your three sets, and if you manage to go just 1 better, then mark that down as a PB too.

Once you see those PBs stacking up in your training diary, it'll show you clearly that you're making solid progress – and give you plenty of fuel for progressing even further in the coming weeks.

Gym Workouts

You'll be continuing with The Three Set Shocker training system for the second consecutive week, followed by a finisher exercise at the end of every session.

There's just one new muscle isolation exercise this week: dumbbell row. This is a pretty straightforward back exercise, and there's a video guide on this one too on my YouTube channel.

Week 4, Workout 1

TRAINING SYSTEM – The Three Set Shocker

EXERCISE	SETS	REPS	REST	WEIGHT	NOTE
Deadlifts	3	6-9	60 secs		
Squats	3	6-9	60 secs		
Barbell curls	3	6-9	60 secs		
Arnie press	3	6-9	60 secs		
Assisted chin-ups	3	6-9	60 secs		
Dumbbell row	3	6-9	60 secs		
Bent over row	3	6-9	60 secs		
FINISHER: Light barbell curls	5	9	**10 secs** (half weight, only 10 secs rest)		

Week 4, Workout 2

TRAINING SYSTEM – The Three Set Shocker

EXERCISE	SETS	REPS	REST	WEIGHT	NOTE
Military press	3	6-9	60 secs		
Bench press	3	6-9	60 secs		
Lat pulldown	3	6-9	60 secs		
Cable row	3	6-9	60 secs		
Assisted chin-ups	3	6-9	60 secs		
Assisted dips	3	6-9	60 secs		
Triceps pushdown	3	6-9	60 secs		
FINISHER: Light military press	**5**	**9**	**10 secs** (half weight, only 10 secs rest)		

Week 4, Workout 3

TRAINING SYSTEM – The Three Set Shocker

EXERCISE	SETS	REPS	REST	WEIGHT	NOTE
Deadlifts	3	6-9	60 secs		
Squats	3	6-9	60 secs		
Barbell curls	3	6-9	60 secs		
Clean & press	3	6-9	60 secs		
Bent over row	3	6-9	60 secs		

Arnie press	3	6-9	60 secs		
Dumbbell row	3	6-9	60 secs		
FINISHER: Light clean & press	5	9	**10 secs** (half weight, only 10 secs rest)		

* Hit the gym 3 times this week and follow along the workouts in your training diary.

* Train 1 day on, 1 day off (such as Mon, Wed, Fri).

* Don't be skipping any workouts!

Nutrition

* Do intermittent fasting Mon-Fri, aiming for a fast of 14-16 hours. Remember, this is easily done by skipping breakfast.

* Relax your diet a little at the weekend. Have a takeaway meal if you like, and the odd treat after working hard in the gym. Remember not to do intermittent fasting at the weekend too.

* Follow the golden rules of clean eating (cut out sugar as much as you can, eat more vegetables and fruit, cook fresh as much as possible, drink enough water each day, beware of the long ingredients list and dodgy additives in foods, and don't microwave your food).

Accountability

* Fill in your gym training diary completely as you go along in the gym. Mark down the weights you lift and the number of repetitions you managed in each set in your diary's notes section. This will give you targets to beat next time around and ensure solid progress.

* Complete a weekly review in your gym diary at the end of the week. Give yourself weekly scores out of 10 for your training, your diet, and your quality of sleep. Then write down one thing that worked really well, one thing you can improve upon, and also jot down how many personal bests you achieved in total for the week.

Positive Habit

* Take 1 step every day this week to reduce the amount of sugar in your diet. Usually have 2 sugars in your tea or coffee? Reduce it to 1 sugar – or drink less tea or coffee and replace it with water. Have some chocolate after your lunch? Swap it for a healthier snack like nuts or fruit.

Chapter 8

Isolation Exercises For Muscle Definition (Week 5)

We're now approaching the halfway stage and the theme for this week is muscle isolation exercises – as we're introducing four new awesome ones this week.

Those exercises are: reverse flyes, which targets the rear shoulder muscles, then deltoid raises which works the front of the shoulders, helping to sculpt a nice round shape.

Next up is the pec deck, a seated machine exercise that targets the chest muscles and also hits the front of the shoulders again. Finally, we're also adding in lying bench curls, which involves doing dumbbell curls for your biceps lying at a slight angle on a bench.

Working the biceps this way brings more muscle fibres into play, sparking more muscle development and better definition. Watch the demonstration videos to get the hang of all four exercises.

Gym Workouts

Let's begin with some good news: there's no finisher exercise this week. Or next week either! The finisher can absolutely floor you after a good weights workout (although that's the idea), but this program is always evolving.

We never want to get stuck in a rut in the gym, and it's important to keep testing your body by continually changing things up.

Week 5, Workout 1

TRAINING SYSTEM – The Three Set Shocker

EXERCISE	SETS	REPS	REST	WEIGHT	NOTE
Squats	3	6-9	60 secs		
Deadlifts	3	6-9	60 secs		
Reverse flyes	3	6-9	60 secs		
Deltoid raises	3	6-9	60 secs		
Assisted chin-ups	3	6-9	60 secs		
Dumbbell row	3	6-9	60 secs		
Lying bench curls	3	6-9	60 secs		
Barbell curls	3	6-9	60 secs		

Week 5, Workout 2

TRAINING SYSTEM – The Three Set Shocker

EXERCISE	SETS	REPS	REST	WEIGHT	NOTE
Dumbbell press	3	6-9	60 secs		
Pec deck	3	6-9	60 secs		
Dumbbell flyes	3	6-9	60 secs		
Assisted dips	3	6-9	60 secs		
Clean & press	3	6-9	60 secs		
Assisted dips	3	6-9	60 secs		
Triceps pushdown	3	6-9	60 secs		
Upright row	3	6-9	60 secs		

Week 5, Workout 3

TRAINING SYSTEM – The Three Set Shocker

EXERCISE	SETS	REPS	REST	WEIGHT	NOTE
Clean & press	3	6-9	60 secs		
Deadlifts	3	6-9	60 secs		
Squats	3	6-9	60 secs		
Lying bench curls	3	6-9	60 secs		
Assisted chin-ups	3	6-9	60 secs		
Bent over row	3	6-9	60 secs		

| Barbell curls | 3 | 6-9 | 60 secs | | |
| Arnie press | 3 | 6-9 | 60 secs | | |

* Hit the gym 3 times this week and follow along the workouts in your training diary.

* Train 1 day on, 1 day off (such as Mon, Wed, Fri).

* Don't be skipping any workouts!

Nutrition

* Do intermittent fasting Mon-Fri, aiming for a fast of 14-16 hours. Remember, this is easily done by skipping breakfast.

* Relax your diet a little at the weekend. Have a takeaway meal if you like, and the odd treat after working hard in the gym. Remember not to do intermittent fasting at the weekend too.

* Follow the golden rules of clean eating (cut out sugar as much as you can, eat more vegetables and fruit, cook fresh as much as possible, drink enough water each day, beware of the long ingredients list and dodgy additives in foods, and don't microwave your food).

Accountability

* Fill in your gym training diary completely as you go along in the gym. Mark down the weights you lift and the number of repetitions you managed in each set in your diary's notes section. This will give you targets to beat next time around and ensure solid progress.

* Complete a weekly review in your gym diary at the end of the week. Give yourself weekly scores out of 10 for your training, your diet, and your quality of sleep. Then write down one thing that worked really well, one thing you can improve upon, and also jot down how many personal bests you achieved in total for the week.

Positive Habit

* Make at least 1 of your workouts an early morning session on an empty stomach. That means getting of bed and heading to the gym to get a good weights workout done before the day has even begun.

I realise this might be tricky if you leave for work early midweek or have young kids, but it's only 1 early session. If you can't manage it midweek, then do it at the weekend.

Choose that early morning workout day and time right now. Don't leave it to chance, schedule it immediately. Then you can get that day off to the best start with a seriously good morning workout, while most other people in your town are still lying in their bed.

Chapter 9

Drop Sets (Week 6)

I don't just want you to be strong. I want you to be fit, healthy and vital.

There's a big misconception that lifting weights is all about muscle and strength. Done correctly, at the right intensity, it also really gets the heart rate up and works the cardiovascular system hard. Just ask anyone who has tried Crossfit for the first time!

The new training system being introduced now in Week 6 requires an increased cardio output; more so than the Three Sets Heavy or Three Set Shocker done up until now.

It's called 'Drop Sets' because you'll be dropping the level of weight after each set. While the weight goes down, the intensity actually goes up because you're only allowed 20-30 secs rest in between each of those sets.

Drop Sets is one of my favourite training systems, so much so that I describe it in my first book Strength Training NOT Bodybuilding', cover it in my sixth 'Fitness Hacking'...and here I am banging on it about it again.

The beauty of this training system is that it speeds up your workouts and you can be finished up in the gym in literally 35-40 mins.

But it's definitely not easier. The idea behind it is that you reduce the weight you're lifting incrementally – but it's the lack of rest between those sets that works you hard and really fatigues the muscles effectively.

Here's how it works in action:

Step 1

Begin set number of any exercise with a fairly heavy weight where you can do between 6-9 reps.

Step 2

Reduce the weight by around 25%, and then quickly begin set number two of the exercise after around 30 secs rest (which is usually just enough time to take the discs off the bar and get started again).

Step 3

Finish set number two and reduce the weight by another 25% (always remembering to lock the safety collars back in place) and then jump straight into your third and final set.

Gym Workouts

Note: there's no finisher exercise again this week. You won't be needing it anyway as Drop Sets are going to do a number on you this week. May God have mercy on your sweet soul.

Week 6, Workout 1

TRAINING SYSTEM – Drop Sets

EXERCISE	SETS	REPS	REST	WEIGHT	NOTE
Squats	3	6-9	30 secs		
Assisted dips	3	6-9	30 secs		
Military press	3	6-9	30 secs		
Reverse flyes	3	6-9	30 secs		
Barbell curls	3	6-9	30 secs		
Assisted chin-ups	3	6-9	30 secs		
Lying bench curls	3	6-9	30 secs		
Cable row	3	6-9	30 secs		

Week 6, Workout 2

TRAINING SYSTEM – Drop Sets

EXERCISE	SETS	REPS	REST	WEIGHT	NOTE
Dumbbell press	3	6-9	30 secs		
Lat pulldown	3	6-9	30 secs		
Pec deck	3	6-9	30 secs		
Assisted dips	3	6-9	30 secs		
Triceps pushdown	3	6-9	30 secs		
Upright row	3	6-9	30 secs		
Cable row	3	6-9	30 secs		
Dumbbell row	3	6-9	30 secs		

Week 6, Workout 3

TRAINING SYSTEM – Drop Sets

EXERCISE	SETS	REPS	REST	WEIGHT	NOTE
Assisted chin-ups	3	6-9	30 secs		
Bench press	3	6-9	30 secs		
Deltoid raises	3	6-9	30 secs		
Arnie press	3	6-9	30 secs		
Dumbbell row	3	6-9	30 secs		
Assisted dips	3	6-9	30 secs		

| Barbell curls | 3 | 6-9 | 30 secs | | |
| Lying bench curls | 3 | 6-9 | 30 secs | | |

* Hit the gym 3 times this week and follow along the workouts in your training diary.

* Train 1 day on, 1 day off (such as Mon, Wed, Fri).

*Don't be skipping any workouts!

Nutrition

* Do intermittent fasting Mon-Fri, aiming for a fast of 14-16 hours. Remember, this is easily done by skipping breakfast.

* Relax your diet a little at the weekend. Have a takeaway meal if you like, and the odd treat after working hard in the gym. Remember not to do intermittent fasting at the weekend too.

* Follow the golden rules of clean eating (cut out sugar as much as you can, eat more vegetables and fruit, cook fresh as much as possible, drink enough water each day, beware of the long ingredients list and dodgy additives in foods, and don't microwave your food).

Accountability

* Fill in your gym training diary completely as you go along in the gym. Mark down the weights you lift and the number of repetitions you managed in each set in your diary's notes section. This will give you targets to beat next time around and ensure solid progress.

* Complete a weekly review in your gym diary at the end of the week. Give yourself weekly scores out of 10 for your training, your diet, and your quality of sleep. Then write down one thing that worked really well, one thing you can improve upon, and also jot down how many personal bests you achieved in total for the week.

Positive Habit

* Get to your bed at a reasonable time every day Mon-Fri and try to get at least seven hours of sleep. Sufficient sleep is so important as this is when your body goes to work to repair and redevelop after your gym workouts.

A restful sleep is also crucial for maintaining good health, said Captain Obvious. But seriously, no perfect diet or expensive supplements can come close to what proper sleep does for your health.

Chapter 10

Creating A Stronger Self Image (Week 7)

This might well be the most important chapter in the book. We're going to look closely at something you may not have expected.

Something that's hugely important, yet is barely talked about in health and fitness.

The very thing that's likely held you back from achieving your fitness goals in the past, and caused you to revert to old bad habits time after time.

I'm talking about the self-image.

The bottom line is: you can work out like a maniac in the gym and stick religiously to a super clean diet...but if you've got a negative self-image you'll struggle to see positive results.

You can reach a certain level of success in changing your bodyshape through perseverance, but if you don't cultivate a strong self-image you'll almost certainly end up back at square one.

We all know someone who has been on yo-yo diets most of their lives. They go to Slimming World or Weight Watchers, lose loads of weight, and then pile it all back on again.

And we all know someone who has tried a gazillion different ways to get fit – jogging, fitness classes or even weight training – and jumped from one thing to another in frustration because they just weren't seeing results. That person might even be you.

In many cases, the problem is not with the fitness program (because other people have clearly had success with it) but the person's own self-image is undermining all their hard efforts with fitness and diet.

Your Self Image Determines What You Can And Can't Achieve

"Our self-image prescribes the limits for the accomplishment of any particular goals."

This is quote by Maxwell Maltz, author of the phenomenal book Psycho-Cybernetics. I've referred to this classic once or twice before in my other fitness books and I don't apologise one bit for doing so again. This stuff is too important.

What is the self-image? This concept is that we all have a particular view of ourselves that is controlled by our mental programs. This self-image then determines your behavior – and what you can and can't achieve.

Ultimately, Psycho-Cybernetics defines the mind-body connection and the self-image as the core of success in attaining personal goals.

This is not widely known at all, but this information has been around since 1960 when Maxwell Maltz first published Psycho-Cybernetics. It's since sold over 30 million copies, and should be essential reading for every human that can read.

There are several techniques described in the book that you can apply in order to improve your self-image and thus create new results in your life.

This is not some think-abundance-and-you'll-be-showered-in-abundance bullshit. There are specific practical steps you can take to help undo unhelpful negative mental programs, and install better ones.

And for the frustrated, self-critical people who feel like they're always taking one step forward and then two steps back with their diet and fitness, well addressing self-image issues may finally be the key to breaking free from all of that.

I'd highly recommend reading this book yourself – as it's potentially life-changing – but for now I'll just cover a few basic lessons from it, and how you can use its wisdom to develop a stronger self-image.

This will be like rocket fuel for achieving your fitness goals, and achieving success in other areas of your life.

Spend 10 mins thinking about what you think about yourself physically.

* What kind of things do you say to yourself?

* Are you often critical of yourself for the shape you're in, or lack of willpower?

* Do you sometimes feel uncomfortable standing in front of the mirror...when that self-critic gets louder in your mind?

* Do you always doubt that you're even capable of achieving the great body and fitness levels you want?

The research done by Maxwell Maltz demonstrated that we can change our long-held negative thought patterns and mental programs that may have been holding us back for years.

You can install new mental programs and develop a brand new, better self-image. It's done through:

* Repeated conscious effort and visualization

* Backed up with positive emotion

* Done continuously for 21 days or more, according to neuroscience research

When I talk about visualization, it's not just a case of thinking positive thoughts about you being superfit and in the greatest shape of your life. **Combining your imagination with positive emotion** is what brings the changes.

Once you begin acting as if you've already achieved what you want, and start feeling like how you would feel when you achieve all of your fitness goals, it sends the right signals to your nervous system — and your subconscious mind does not know the difference.

Doing this on repeat for at least 21 days can bring a massive shift and shape a whole new self-image. This might sound like airy fairy stuff to you, but it's real and it's been proven to work.

You just have to put in the conscious effort and do it repeatedly to create the desired changes in your self-image.

Gym Workouts

Four new exercises are introduced this week: quad machine (legs); hamstring machine (legs), narrow grip bench press (triceps), and the mighty assisted pull-ups, a tough compound exercise that works your back, shoulders, arms and core hard.

For the second week running, you'll be working with the Drop Sets system, so remember to decrease the weight by 25% after each set, and take no more than 30 secs rest in between those sets.

Week 7, Workout 1

TRAINING SYSTEM – Drop Sets

EXERCISE	SETS	REPS	REST	WEIGHT	NOTE
Bench press	3	6-9	30 secs		
Reverse flyes	3	6-9	30 secs		
Dumbbell flyes	3	6-9	30 secs		
Assisted dips	3	6-9	30 secs		
Narrow grip bench press	3	6-9	30 secs		
Military press	3	6-9	30 secs		
Overhead rope ext.	3	6-9	30 secs		
Triceps pushdown	3	6-9	30 secs		

Week 7, Workout 2

TRAINING SYSTEM – Drop Sets

EXERCISE	SETS	REPS	REST	WEIGHT	NOTE
Squats	3	6-9	30 secs		

Quad machine	3	6-9	30 secs		
Hamstring machine	3	6-9	30 secs		
Deadlifts	3	6-9	30 secs		
Upright row	3	6-9	30 secs		
Deltoid raises	3	6-9	30 secs		
Bent over row	3	6-9	30 secs		
Lat pulldown	3	6-9	30 secs		

Week 7, Workout 3

TRAINING SYSTEM – Drop Sets

EXERCISE	SETS	REPS	REST	WEIGHT	NOTE
Dumbbell press	3	6-9	30 secs		
Assisted pull-ups	3	6-9	30 secs		
Dumbbell flyes	3	6-9	30 secs		
Assisted chin-ups	3	6-9	30 secs		
Assisted dips	3	6-9	30 secs		
Clean & press	3	6-9	30 secs		
Upright row	3	6-9	30 secs		
Overhead rope ext.	3	6-9	30 secs		

* Hit the gym 3 times this week and follow along the workouts in your training diary.

* Train 1 day on, 1 day off (such as Mon, Wed, Fri).

* Don't be skipping any workouts!

Nutrition

* Do intermittent fasting Mon-Fri, aiming for a fast of 14-16 hours. Remember, this is easily done by skipping breakfast.

* Relax your diet a little at the weekend. Have a takeaway meal if you like, and the odd treat after working hard in the gym. Remember not to do intermittent fasting at the weekend too.

* Follow the golden rules of clean eating – you know them well enough by now.

Accountability

* Fill in your gym training diary completely as you go along in the gym. Mark down the weights you lift and the number of repetitions you managed in each set in your diary's notes section. This will give you targets to beat next time around and ensure solid progress.

* Complete a weekly review in your gym diary at the end of the week. Give yourself weekly scores out of 10 for your training, your diet, and your quality of sleep. Then write down one thing that worked really well, one thing you can improve upon, and also jot down how many personal bests you achieved in total for the week.

Positive Habit

* If there's one really positive habit to implement this week that could have a huge impact on your life, it's for you to buy Psycho-Cybernetics. You can buy a copy on the Amazon website.

Chapter 11

It's Time To Burn (Week 8)

If you haven't been feeling the burn in your muscles during your workouts, you definitely will this week.

That's because we're introducing a new training system that I call 'The Slow Burner'. The idea behind this is that you do 2 x heavy sets of each exercise with a normal rest period of 60 secs, but then for the final set you're focusing on going slowly for 4-5 secs.

This deliberate slower motion is implemented in the second part of each exercise, putting the muscles under tension and creates the burning feeling.

There are two parts to every exercise – concentric (also known as positive) and eccentric (also referred to as negative).

Concentric is when you contract the muscles and make them shorter, like when you bend down doing squats or squeeze your biceps as you curl a barbell upwards.

Eccentric/negative is the lowering part of the movement where you extend and lengthen the muscles.

It's this part where you're going to do slower, more controlled repetitions...for around 4-5 secs instead of just 1 or 2.

For example, I would usually do the military press with around 50kg and do normal repetitions of pressing the bar above my head and then lowering back down again.

During a slow burner set, I would press 25kg and the second lowering part of the movement would be done more slowly for around 4-5 secs, and then I'd push back up quickly and more forcefully again. This is done for 6-9 reps.

Or if I was doing squats, usually I'd lower my body down within 1 second before springing back up again with the weight. In the slow burner set, I'd half the overall weight and then bend my knees more slowly so that it takes 4-5 secs before I reach the squatting position. Then I'd press back up again quickly to get into the starting position, and repeat for 6-9 reps.

Just so we're clear, here's how the Slow Burner works...

* Do set 1 as normal, lifting a heavy weight where you can complete between 6 and 9 reps.

* Then take 60 secs rest.

* If you managed 9 reps in set 1 then increase the weight for set 2 and if you couldn't complete 6 reps then of course you'll have to reduce the weight slightly. You know the drill by now.

* After completing set 2 take another 60 secs rest.

* Then cut the overall weight by half for set number three and complete those slower, more controlled repetitions in the negative part of your exercises.

Gym Workouts

Just one new exercise along with the new training system this week, and that's dumbbell lunges. This is a great exercise that targets your glutes and legs.

Week 8, Workout 1

TRAINING SYSTEM – The Slow Burner

EXERCISE	SETS	REPS	REST	WEIGHT	NOTE
Bench press	3	6-9	60 secs		
Assisted pull-ups	3	6-9	60 secs		
Dumbbell lunges	3	6-9	60 secs		
Dumbbell flyes	3	6-9	60 secs		
Assisted dips	3	6-9	60 secs		
Pec deck	3	6-9	60 secs		

Narrow grip bench press	3	6-9	60 secs
Overhead rope ext.	3	6-9	60 secs
FINISHER: Light pec	5	9	**10 secs** deck (Half usual weight, only 10 secs rest)

Week 8, Workout 2

TRAINING SYSTEM – The Slow Burner

EXERCISE	SETS	REPS	REST	WEIGHT	NOTE
Squats	3	6-9	60 secs		
Hamstring machine	3	6-9	60 secs		
Quad machine	3	6-9	60 secs		
Military press	3	6-9	60 secs		
Bent over row	3	6-9	60 secs		
Arnie press	3	6-9	60 secs		
Cable row	3	6-9	60 secs		
FINISHER: Squats	5	9	**10 secs** (Half usual weight, only secs secs rest)		

Week 8, Workout 3

TRAINING SYSTEM – The Slow Burner

EXERCISE	SETS	REPS	REST	WEIGHT	NOTE
Assisted chin-ups	3	6-9	60 secs		
Bench press	3	6-9	60 secs		
Dumbbell flyes	3	6-9	60 secs		
Dumbbell lunges	3	6-9	60 secs		
Assisted dips	3	6-9	60 secs		
Triceps pushdown	3	6-9	60 secs		
Reverse flyes	3	6-9	60 secs		
Overhead rope ext.	3	6-9	60 secs		
FINISHER: Bench press	5	9	**10 secs** (Half usual weight, only 10 secs rest)		

* Hit the gym 3 times this week and follow along the workouts in your training diary.

* Train 1 day on, 1 day off (such as Mon, Wed, Fri).

* Don't be skipping any workouts!

Nutrition

* Do intermittent fasting Mon-Fri, aiming for a fast of 14-16 hours. Remember, this is easily done by skipping breakfast.

* Relax your diet a little at the weekend. Have a takeaway meal if you like, and the odd treat after working hard in the gym. Remember not to do intermittent fasting at the weekend too.

* Stick to the golden rules of clean eating.

Accountability

* Fill in your gym training diary completely as you go along in the gym. Mark down the weights you lift and the number of repetitions you managed in each set in your diary's notes section. This will give you targets to beat next time around and ensure solid progress.

* Complete a weekly review in your gym diary at the end of the week. Give yourself weekly scores out of 10 for your training, your diet, and your quality of sleep. Then write down one thing that worked really well, one thing you can improve upon, and also jot down how many personal bests you achieved in total for the week.

Positive Habit

* Let's return our attention to your diet again. I want you to cook three new healthy dinners at home this week using fresh ingredients. Something you don't usually have. Make a big batch and then keep leftovers for lunch the next day – a useful habit for eating healthily.

Forget the excuses that you can't cook, or don't have time. Google some new healthy recipes, hit the supermarket for the ingredients, and get cooking on at least three different nights this week.

Chapter 12

Rising To A Whole New Level (Week 9)

You're nearly there! It's the penultimate week of the program – and that means we need to step things up and rise to a whole new level!

By this point you'll undoubtedly be much stronger than you were in week 1, and you'll be super confident in the gym. After doing eight solid weeks of training as laid out in this program, you'll be way past the novice stage.

As it's all about steady progress and continually pushing yourself with the Be Your Own PT program, let's take it up a notch.

As you know, we quite like personal bests around here. So, for week 9 you might imagine I'd want you to hit 9 new personal bests. Let's just go for a nice round number and make it 10.

Make this your best week yet and hit a **total of 10 new PBs** over the course of your 3 workouts. Remember to mark them up in your gym diary as you work through each session.

So, let's take things to the next level this week. Those 10 personal bests are a big ask, but think about how amazing you'll feel once you start seeing all those PBs piling up in your training diary.

Remember, it's 10 in total. That could mean 3 in gym session 1, another 4 in session 2, and a further 3 in your third session. Just push yourself hard as there's only two weeks left of the program remaining.

Gym Workouts

Deltoid raises is a new muscle isolation exercise thrown in the mix this week. This is a straightforward exercise where stand up straight with a dumbbell in each hand resting against your thighs, and you then raise your arms up straight in front of you.

This movement targets the front of the shoulders and is one of the easiest dumbbell exercises you can do, technique wise. Check out deltoid raises in the Exercises Guide Index at the end of the book.

Week 9, Workout 1

TRAINING SYSTEM – The Slow Burner

EXERCISE	SETS	REPS	REST	WEIGHT	NOTE
Bench press	3	6-9	60 secs		
Assisted pull-ups	3	6-9	60 secs		
Pec deck	3	6-9	60 secs		
Dumbbell row	3	6-9	60 secs		
Assisted dips	3	6-9	60 secs		

Exercise	Sets	Reps	Rest	Weight	Note
Bent over row	3	6-9	60 secs		
Overhead rope ext.	3	6-9	60 secs		
Triceps pushdown	3	6-9	60 secs		
FINISHER: Bench	5	9	**10 secs** press (Half usual weight, only 10 secs rest)		

Week 9, Workout 2

TRAINING SYSTEM – The Slow Burner

EXERCISE	SETS	REPS	REST	WEIGHT	NOTE
Squats	3	6-9	60 secs		
Quad machine	3	6-9	60 secs		
Hamstring machine	3	6-9	60 secs		
Upright row	3	6-9	60 secs		
Military press	3	6-9	60 secs		
Assisted pull-ups	3	6-9	60 secs		
Arnie press	3	6-9	60 secs		
Deltoid raises	3	6-9	60 secs		
FINISHER: Squats	5	9	**10 secs** (Half usual weight, only 10 secs rest)		

Week 9, Workout 3

TRAINING SYSTEM – The Slow Burner

EXERCISE	SETS	REPS	REST	WEIGHT	NOTE
Military press	3	6-9	60 secs		
Assisted chin-ups	3	6-9	60 secs		
Dumbbell press	3	6-9	60 secs		
Dumbbell flyes	3	6-9	60 secs		
Assisted dips	3	6-9	60 secs		
Triceps pushdown	3	6-9	60 secs		
Lat pulldown	3	6-9	60 secs		
Overhead rope ext.	3	6-9	60 secs		
FINISHER: Dumbbell press	5	9	**10 secs** (Half usual weight, only 10 secs rest)		

* Hit the gym 3 times this week and follow along the workouts in your training diary.

* Train 1 day on, 1 day off (such as Mon, Wed, Fri).

* Don't be skipping any workouts!

Nutrition

* Do intermittent fasting Mon-Fri, aiming for a fast of 14-16 hours. Remember, this is easily done by skipping breakfast.

* Relax your diet a little at the weekend. Have a takeaway meal if you like, and the odd treat after working hard in the gym. Remember not to do intermittent fasting at the weekend too.

* Keep following the golden rules of clean eating.

Accountability

* Fill in your gym training diary completely as you go along in the gym. Mark down the weights you lift and the number of repetitions you managed in each set in your diary's notes section. This will give you targets to beat next time around and ensure solid progress.

* Complete a weekly review in your gym diary at the end of the week. Give yourself weekly scores out of 10 for your training, your diet, and your quality of sleep. Then write down one thing that worked really well, one thing you can improve upon, and also jot down how many personal bests you achieved in total for the week.

Positive Habit

* A slightly-unusual habit this week, but one that's geared towards improving your health. Every morning this week start your day by drinking a pint of lemon water.

Squeeze the juice of half a lemon into the glass, half fill with cold water, and then top up with boiling water to make a nice warm refreshing drink.

As well as hydrating for the day ahead, lemon water has numerous health benefits including detoxification, aiding your digestive system, healthier skin. It also boosts your immune system as it's a good source of vitamin C.

Chapter 13

The Final Push...And Celebrations (Week 10)

We're now on the final straight – so let's round off 10 weeks of hard work in style.

Make this your best week yet, and enjoy it. Remember it's a challenge in the gym, not a struggle.

And at the end of this week, it's time to celebrate. No point in busting your ass for 10 weeks if you can't properly enjoy reaching the finish line.

Gym Workouts

No new exercise on this final week, just a spanking mix of those monster compound exercises and all the excellent muscle isolation moves that have been filtered into the program as the weeks have gone on.

Sticking with The Slow Burner for the third consecutive week, let's make these last three workouts really count.

Week 10, Workout 1

TRAINING SYSTEM – The Slow Burner

EXERCISE	SETS	REPS	REST	WEIGHT	NOTE
Squats	3	6-9	60 secs		
Lat pulldown	3	6-9	60 secs		
Bent over row	3	6-9	60 secs		
Assisted pull-ups	3	6-9	60 secs		
Military press	3	6-9	60 secs		
Upright row	3	6-9	60 secs		
Arnie press	3	6-9	60 secs		
Deltoid raises	3	6-9	60 secs		
FINISHER: Military press	5	9	**10 secs** (Half usual weight, only 10 secs rest)		

Week 10, Workout 2

TRAINING SYSTEM – The Slow Burner

EXERCISE	SETS	REPS	REST	WEIGHT	NOTE
Assisted chin-ups	3	6-9	60 secs		
Bench press	3	6-9	60 secs		

Cable row	3	6-9	60 secs		
Dumbbell flyes	3	6-9	60 secs		
Assisted dips	3	6-9	60 secs		
Bent over row	3	6-9	60 secs		
Overhead rope ext.	3	6-9	60 secs		
Triceps pushdown	3	6-9	60 secs		
FINISHER: Cable row	5	9	10 secs (Half usual weight, only 10 secs rest)		

Week 10, Workout 3

TRAINING SYSTEM – The Slow Burner

EXERCISE	SETS	REPS	REST	WEIGHT	NOTE
Squats	3	6-9	60 secs		
Dumbbell lunges	3	6-9	60 secs		
Quad leg machine	3	6-9	60 secs		
Hamstring machine	3	6-9	60 secs		
Assisted chin-ups	3	6-9	60 secs		
Bent over row	3	6-9	60 secs		
Arnie press	3	6-9	60 secs		

Lat pulldown	3	6-9	60 secs		
FINISHER: Quad machine	5	9	**10 secs** ((Half usual weight, only 10 secs rest)		

* Hit the gym 3 times this week and follow along the workouts in your training diary.

* Train 1 day on, 1 day off (such as Mon, Wed, Fri).

* Don't be skipping any workouts!

Nutrition

* Do intermittent fasting Mon-Fri, aiming for a fast of 14-16 hours. Remember, this is easily done by skipping breakfast.

* Relax your diet a little at the weekend. Have a takeaway meal if you like, and the odd treat after working hard in the gym. Remember not to do intermittent fasting at the weekend too.

* Follow the golden rules of clean eating.

Accountability

* Fill in your gym training diary completely as you go along in the gym. Mark down the weights you lift and the number of repetitions you managed in each set in your diary's notes section. This will give you targets to beat next time around and ensure solid progress.

* Complete a weekly review in your gym diary at the end of the week. Give yourself weekly scores out of 10 for your training, your diet, and your quality of sleep. Then write down one thing that worked really well, one thing you can improve upon, and also jot down how many personal bests you achieved in total for the week.

Positive Habit

There's one very important task that I want you to complete for this week...

And that's to treat yourself to a meal at a nice restaurant, or your favourite takeaway meal. Maybe even buy yourself some new clothes to fit that stronger, leaner body of yours.

I'm saying this because you'll have worked hard as hell in this Be Your Own PT program and now it's time to celebrate. You've earned it, now enjoy it.

PART THREE
SUCCESS STORIES

Chapter 14

From A 310lbs Mountain Of Flab...To A Rock Solid Gym Machine

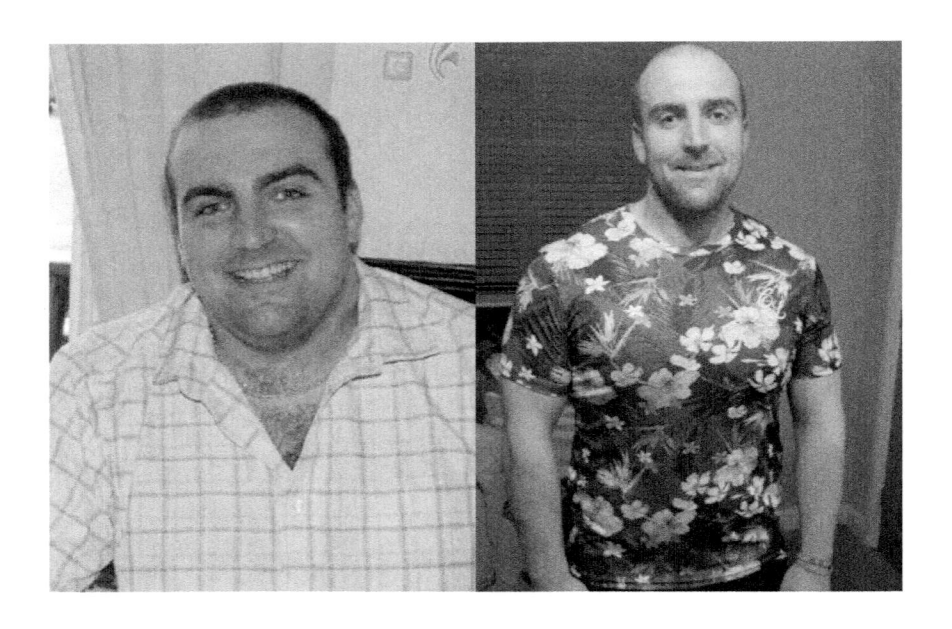

You know someone's serious about becoming superfit when they tell you they've climbed Mount Kilimanjaro.

John Hick spent many months in the gym building up his strength and endurance to conquer the monster mountain, which is almost 20,000ft high and generally takes hikers 5-7 days to summit.

The 31-year-old and a group of fellow trekkers made it to the top at the end of December 2019, before heading home safely to England to start 2020 on a high.

But the ice had barely melted on John's boots before he gave himself another mountainous challenge: losing two stone over the next 10 weeks.

John had always been "quite a big chap". His words, not mine.

His weight ballooned to 22 stone (almost 310lbs) at his heaviest, but he'd managed to shed around five stone mainly through walking and indoor climbing. For the previous three years John's weight fluctuated between 17 stone and 18 stone, with John always struggling to find a diet and fitness approach to stick with.

Atkins diet, juicing, eating just 1,000 calories a day...John had tried it all to lose fat and get in better shape.

"I've been trying to lose weight and tone up for five years," said John. "I have tried fad diets and cardio plans and various other exercise plans but with no consistency.

"I left other fitness plans behind because most of them were inconsistent and not sustainable in the long term.

"I decided to take up weight training when I learned about it being an easier way to lose weight via increased metabolism instead of cardio workouts.

"I never wanted to become a massive bodybuilder type but discovered that weightlifting was more about strength, not becoming a meat head, which is a massive misconception."

It was this realisation that drew John to the first book in my series, *Strength Training NOT Bodybuilding*.

"I loved this approach towards fitness and the fact that your focus was on strength, not size," John told me.

Up until that point John had been advised to eat 1200 calories per day – a ridiculously low amount for a man of his size – whilst burning 1000 calories doing cardio.

"It just wasn't sustainable in any form," said John. "I'd been up and down with my weight for a few years and needed a program that would send me in the right direction for good.

"I wanted to lose two stone in a healthy way, and make sure that I kept the weight off this time."

Why John Was Primed For Some Great Results

As I mentioned before, I asked everyone who showed an interest in signing up for the Be Your Own PT program to fill out an online application form.

I wasn't being an asshole, I was simply wanting to make sure I didn't waste any of their time and they didn't waste any of mine. You see, there's a big difference between saying you want to get in great shape – and actually putting in 10 weeks' worth of effort and achieving it.

With John, my bullshit-o-meter did not indicate any red flags. Infact, I knew he was primed for some great results based on what he told me.

"My problems in the past have been with weekends and booze. I assure you, 2020 is not going to be the same," wrote John.

"Motivation is without a doubt NOT my problem. If I am interested in something, I do it 100%. If I am not interested it's 0%. There's no middle ground with me, I will give you my all.

"2020 will bring me the results I desire, I have never been more certain."

I didn't need any more convincing. John was clearly right up for the challenge, and I was excited to steer him in the right direction, particularly as he'd been so frustrated for so long with all of these crappy fad diets.

None of these diets are sustainable, just as John found out the hard way. There was no need to cut out carbs with the Atkins Diet, drive himself nuts with a juicing only diet plan, or turn himself into a wreck eating just 1,200 calories per day – while burning 1,000 calories doing cardio.

Following that kind of extreme calorie cutting long term will inevitably lead to weakness, fatigue, hormone imbalances, and various other health complications. A seriously bad trade-off just to lose some weight.

This is why my approach of intermittent fasting combined with weight training is so manageable for people like John. It means they can eat a sufficient amount of food each day without sweating about crazy calorie targets.

It also means they're not left starving, feeling weak, or trying to muster up some more willpower just to keep going.

And unlike the Atkins Diet, or any other restrictive diet, no foods are completely banned in the Be Your Own PT program. All I ask is that people follow my clean eating guidelines Monday-Friday, and then relax their diet at the weekend – without going crazy.

It's common sense. It's enjoyable. Most importantly, it can be maintained. After three years of yo-yo dieting and fluctuating between the 16 stone and 18 stone mark, John just wanted a balanced, easier approach.

My bullshit-o-meter was right. It rarely lets me down. John stuck to the promises he made about working his ass off, and within a couple of weeks the results were showing.

"Down 3lbs this week, feeling great…"

"Managed another 4 personal bests, loved the workouts this week…"

These were text messages John was sending my way, and I was buzzing to see him thrive on a training and diet plan he could enjoy. Health and fitness should be challenging, but it should always leave you satisfied and hungry to keep pushing on, rather than having a constant willpower battle.

Much Lighter, Much Stronger, Much Leaner

The timing of the Be Your Own PT program was almost perfect as the recruits were on their final workouts of Week 10 when the world basically went into lockdown due to coronavirus.

Gyms were closed and we were told to stay indoors. But by this time John had already achieved amazing results with the program, and then bought a home weights set so he could maintain them until his gym reopened.

"I've lost almost two stones," said John. "I feel much stronger, look much leaner, and my shoulders look amazing! This is also a much better approach to diet, and one that I can stick with in the future.

"The top three things I enjoyed most about Be Your Own PT were having a training diary with all my workouts, having the community support on WhatsApp, and always pushing myself for PBs.

"The community on WhatsApp made a massive difference. I've always done training on my own in the past, but this time around I've found it a lot easier with friends to turn to and someone there to ask for advice.

"I'll always continue with some form of weight training as part of my workouts now. I feel there is so much more benefit compared to cardio workouts.

"For anyone else in my situation looking to lose weight as well as gain muscle, I would highlight to them that weight training increases metabolism, which in turn does so much more good than under-eating and a fuck load of cardio."

Chapter 15

Athlete Finds The Strength To Get Back To The Top

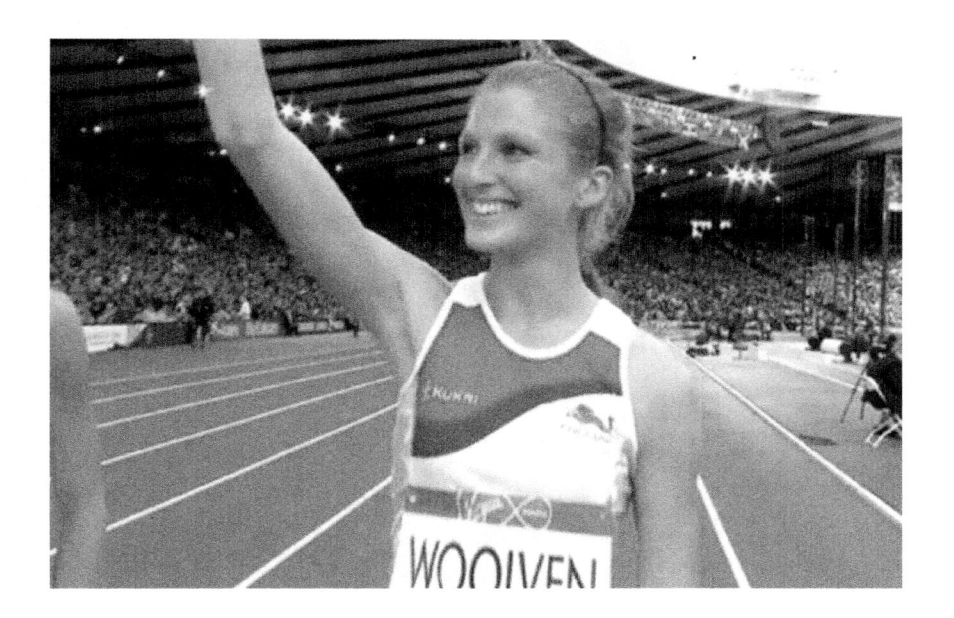

Pippa Woolven's eyes lit up with colour as she gazed around the stadium packed with 50,000 people.

Those crowds locked their eyes on Pippa and the other elite level athletes, while millions more around the world were tuning in through their TVs.

It was the summer of 2014. The location was Glasgow, and the event...the Commonwealth Games. Aged just 20 years old, Pippa was representing her country in the 3,000m steeplechase event.

Proudly wearing her white and red kit, Pippa had already achieved the dream before a gun was sounded. For she was representing England, just like both her parents and three older siblings in various sports, and this was on a huge stage.

"The atmosphere was absolutely amazing, and I'll never forget the feeling of walking out to 50,000 spectators," said Pippa, who lives in Buckinghamshire, near London. "Competing at the 2014 Commonwealth Games is also where I met my partner of five years, Rich."

While the three Kenyan athletes who were tipped as favourites claimed gold, silver and bronze, Pippa put on a blistering performance, recording a personal best time of 9 mins, 47 secs.

Over the last six years, Pippa has also competed in a World Championships event, and won a team silver medal at the European Cross-Country Championships in the Netherlands in 2018.

For all the highs, every athlete must experience lows.

For Pippa that came in early 2019 when she suffered a serious foot injury which derailed her track season for the rest of the year.

All she could do was light training and had to avoid her passion of middle distance running while awaiting surgery.

Weight training had always been in the background, with a couple of light strength and conditioning gym sessions per week to complement her full-on cardio efforts.

But Pippa had never prioritised working on her strength. Endurance, stamina, and shaving milliseconds off her best running times were naturally always at the forefront.

That was all on the backburner after the injury, while Pippa's dream of making the 2020 Tokyo Olympics lay in pieces. The whole situation would test Pippa's resolve, and mental toughness.

Many would have crumbled; gone to a dark place. Instead, Pippa's competitive instinct kicked in and her solution to getting back on track was doing what she knew best.

"It was time for a new challenge," said Pippa. "I decided to see how much strength and fitness I could develop through weight training alone.

"As they say, 'if you change nothing then nothing changes' and I was keen for a change."

This was indeed a complete change in direction for the woman who had been obsessed with running ever since she won an annual cross-country race at primary school.

That day was the first time she'd beaten her older sisters at anything – so Pippa quickly joined a local running club.

There were plenty of positive signs of huge achievements in sport, especially when Pippa won the English Schools National Championships in her late teens.

Following a full athletics scholarship at Florida State University in America, Pippa returned home to start a career with the National Trust heritage organisation whilst competing for Great Britain.

Training at an elite level was always full-on. It required one or two running sessions per day, plus conditioning work in the gym and periods of rest in between. Every lifestyle choice she made wasgearedtowards being the best athlete she could be.

Pippa said: "The highs would include just feeling in peak physical fitness - full of energy and limitless, there is nothing like it! The lows come with illness, injury or anything that came between me and my goals.

"When you invest so much in a sport and a particular lifestyle, it can wreak havoc on your sense of identity and self-worth when you're no longer able to continue.

"Ultimately though, I've come to learn that effort, competitiveness and movement are all aspects of sport that can be redirected when the inevitable illnesses or injuries strike."

Turning her attention to weight training, Pippa picked up my book Strength Training For Women. She then quickly came to the conclusion that her weights workouts had been "aimless and lacklustre", and needed some serious attention.

"I was always reluctant to lift too much weight because of the common misconceptions surrounding muscle mass and becoming 'bulky'," explained Pippa. "As an endurance athlete, I always stuck to a high number of reps, using light weights and kept recovery time to a minimum.

"In hindsight, I was just adding another aerobic session into my weekly routine, when power and strength was what I needed most.

"When I was still dealing with the particularly stubborn foot injury, I signed up for the Be Your Own PT program and discovered what *real* weight training was."

As expected, Pippa was laser-focused and motivated. She was mastering exercises she'd never done before and was enjoying her new weight training approach. Yet, I noticed a few weeks into the program that her progress had slowed up a bit.

I discovered that there were two things holding Pippa back in the gym:

#1 - A reluctance or hesitation to increase the weight and push herself hard enough.

#2 – Insufficient recovery following workouts.

Those two problems went hand in hand. A few weeks into the program, Pippa was trying to resume her running as her foot began to heal. She'd clock up several miles on the same day she was lifting weights.

This simply wasn't going to work if she wanted to increase her strength and improve her performance in the gym.

With weight training gym sessions in this program there's an all-over body workout approach, and the aim is to gradually increase the weights level and intensity to really fatigue the muscles.

What should come next is good nutrition, followed by sufficient rest to allow those muscles to repair and develop. But by throwing in extended runs just a few hours later, Pippa was interfering with the repair and muscle development process.

It meant that she was limiting progress in the program because her body was being overworked. Recovery is extremely important. The hard work is done in the gym, but your body grows and develops when you're sleeping.

Train Hard, Rest Well

So, we came to a compromise. The weight training and running would be done on alternate days, and I also recommended that Pippa take some supplements including ZMA (zinc, magnesium and vitamin B6) and magnesium oil to help get a deep restful sleep after her weights workouts for proper recovery.

A beautiful balance was struck between both sporting disciplines and Pippa came to realise the importance of giving your body more time to recover from intense workouts. Sleep and supplementation playing a huge role in this, of course.

Guess what happened? Pippa's strength levels took off, weights increased, and she began racking up personal best after personal best for tough exercises such as pull-ups and deadlifts.

I could see Pippa's enjoyment grow with each workout, and she really stepped it up a level to finish the last few weeks on a high. Looking, feeling, and performing at her best.

"Now I've learned the importance of lifting heavier weights, maximising recovery, and how less is often more," said Pippa.

"I've come to learn the benefits of true 'strength training' and how quickly the benefits translate into speed on the track.

"Vainly, I was also a little put off by the common misconceptions of lifting heavier weights translating into becoming overly muscular and then carrying around more weight than absolutely necessary for my running. Another myth that has been busted by Marc!"

Benefits Of The Be Your Own PT Program

Earlier in the book I highlighted a list of unexpected benefits that you and others can experience by committing yourself properly to a weight training program like this one.

Remember, it's not all about aesthetics and having the perfect body. There's so much more to gain. I asked Pippa to list the main benefits she got from her 10 weeks of dedication to weight training. She said:

* Increased confidence in my ability to use previously-avoided gym equipment.

* Increased faith in my ability to lift heavy weights - the only limit is the mind.

* Better body composition – more lean muscle mass.

* Increased motivation to hit the gym since I now realise I don't need to spend hours in there.

* Far greater understanding about what I'm doing and why I'm doing it – huge motivator.

* A sense of structure and direction –particularlyimportant for those starting out.

* A fantastic resource with Marc coaching as you continue learning from via his weekly updates.

Despite being an international elite athlete, Pippa admitted she lacked confidence at the beginning of the weight training program when doing new exercises and trying out new pieces of equipment in the gym.

Pippa said: "This was relatively easy to overcome with the exercise demo videos and reassurance from some of the others in the WhatsApp group that they were experiencing the same. "At times I felt impatient with my progress when other people in the group seemed to be doing so well. But eventually I caught up and came to understand how everyone's rate of progression is different and you can't expect miracles right away.

"Some days – often due to hormones – I didn't feel able to give my all or achieve any PBs. By the end of the program I had come to accept that every day isn't going to be your best performance, but every day can be your best effort.

"As an athlete who competes in a relatively individual sport it's been wonderful to share something with a 'team' of others striving towards the same goal."

A return to international level running is on the cards for Pippa, however weight training will still play a part in her weekly fitness routine and she now has a much more effective approach to developing strength.

"It's amazing to see how much can be achieved in just 10 weeks," said Pippa. "Weight training has taught me that even things you never imagined succeeding at are possible when you have a goal and direction."

Chapter 16

A Woman's Decades-Long Fitness Search Is Over

"I spent the majority of my life being a 'thin fat' person."

I was confused when Laurel Jenson first told me this. It took my brain a couple of seconds to figure out what she meant.

Then she followed up with: "I mean that while I've always been lean, I've never had much muscle tone."

But God loves a trier – and Laurel certainly tried plenty to get fit and tone up.

Sporting a pair of colourful leg-warmers and working out to a Jane Fonda VHS tape in her living room. That was Laurel's fitness plan of attack in the late 70s.

In the 80s, it was aerobics classes bouncing around to tunes by California rockers Huey Lewis and the News.

"Seriously, there was a whole lot of jumping around trying to look cute in leotards and sweatbands back then," said Laurel.

In the 90s, she joined an all-women's "fitness spa" where everything was pink and beautiful. Superfit and super-judgemental girls took Laurel's measurements and created a special fitness plan just for her.

All glamour, perfectionism, and comparing themselves to one another. The so-called fitness spa was swiftly ditched…and it was onto something else.

"Then I joined a Gold's Gym," said Laurel. "That was also short-lived because I was too intimidated by all the meatheads lifting and grunting.

"I remember that I paid for a fitness trainer at one point too. It was so evident that he did not want to train a girl that I never went back."

The millennium came around and Laurel went back to her yoga roots for her next health and fitness focus. Then she threw in some hiking, power walking, some more aerobics, jazzercize, and occasionally a spot of running.

Laurel said: "I still do yoga, and I still hike and walk, but running? I hate running! As you can see, this has been a decades long journey or quest, if you will.

"It wasn't that I disliked any of the others, I have fond memories of my aerobics classes. At the time they were fun."

Working as a flight attendant, the California woman had a chance chat with one of her cabin crew colleagues about health and fitness. Her co-worker was a follower of Tosca Reno, a health guru and author who is a big advocate of weight training.

"She was changing her body through weightlifting and she looked amazing," said Laurel. "So, me being me impulsive by nature, I raced to Barnes and Noble and bought one of her books and joined a local gym.

"I knew that I wasn't going to bulk up. My biggest barrier was my confidence."

Later, Laurel came across my book Strength Training for Women, which helps women overcome the biggest mental blocks women have to getting started lifting weights.

"I loved how the book addressed the concerns that many women have," said Laurel. "Specifically, the insecurities when walking into the weight section. The words captured my feelings.

"The book made it so simple. From the 3 sets of 6-9 reps, maintaining good form, increasing weight when you can do 9 reps, and eatingclean. It's a can't fail system."

In previous stints at the gym, Laurel admitted she made common mistakes that held her back. These included using too many gym machines, instead of doing barbell and dumbbell exercises.

She would also set those machines to a low weights level and do a high number of repetitions, rather than increasing the weight and doing fewer repetitions as I preach in all my strength training books.

While she still had to learn the correct technique for all these new barbell and dumbbell exercises and develop her confidence in the gym, Laurel had a few other areas to focus on.

Now aged 57, she wanted a training system that would finally help her tone up – and strengthen her body to protect her from a health issue that ran in the family.

"I've been thin fat for so long and it was fine when I was in my 20s, but when you hit your 50s?" said Laurel.

"I'll just leave it at that. I dreaded looking in the mirror, shopping for clothes, trying on bathing suits etc.

"Also, my grandmother had osteoporosis, and I was concerned about bone density and strength as I aged.

"I also wanted to focus on strength training because I would not be into a fitness class at this stage of the game. I think that they just didn't 'click' with me. I never felt a thrill of accomplishment. There wasn't a mental challenge."

A challenge was exactly what Laurel got when she signed up to the Be Your Own PT group coaching program. With the aim to always increase repetitions and gradually increase the weight, Laurel was continually improving upon her gym performance.

Sending her completed gym training diary to me on a Sunday, I'd regularly see high scores, such as 8/10 or 9/10, for how well she'd trained in the gym, and how her nutrition had gone that week.

It was clear that she was thriving with the workouts structure, training diary approach, and the all-important accountability we covered earlier.

Week after week, I'd see "PB" after "PB" jotted in Laurel's training diary as she pushed herself, increased her gym confidence, and her motivation levels skyrocketed.

Even when Laurel was going from hotel to hotel with her flight attendant job, she sought out the hotel gym and was keeping up with her three workouts per week. Some gym had limited equipment, yet Laurel found workarounds to ensure she continued her steady progress.

Stronger Than She Ever Imagined

The highlight came around week 7 when Laurel completed her first chin-up without any assistance. By the end of the program, she was doing a total of seven bodyweight chin-ups over 3 sets, and similar numbers with pull-ups – which are even more difficult.

There are very few women in their 50s who can do this. In fact, there are few women who can do this at any age.

But Laurel was so focused on developing her strength and building that bone density that she achieved more than she ever thought she would.

It just proves that, with the right plan and commitment to that plan, any woman or man can become significantly stronger and achieve their fitness goals in as little as 10 weeks.

I asked Laurel what were the biggest benefits she experienced at the end of the 10 weeks, and she replied: "My self confidence in the gym, feeling stronger, leaner, having more energy and a clear mind."

Despite this, it wasn't all plain sailing. Laurel admitted that some weeks proved difficult as life got in the way – and excuses filtered into her mind.

"It was tough managing to find a gym sometimes while travelling," she said. "I had to do a lot of improvising. But I knew that I couldn't let my coach down – I had to find a way to make a way!

"Seriously, it would have been very easy to say 'oh well, not this week', but I just wasn't going to let myself down.

"Having a group of like-minded individuals alongside me was so helpful. The positivity and encouragement was amazing. I doubt that I would have been as successful if I had 'gone it alone'.

"And yes, I'm going to stick with weight training. I absolutely love going to the gym. I am a much more confident person. I'm a lot stronger and feel great. I'll definitely continue with my training. I've created new positive habits.

"If you're new to weight training and considering getting started, I would say 'DO IT!' The results that you are going to get will astound you."

Chapter 17

Muscle & Strength Without A Military-Style Approach

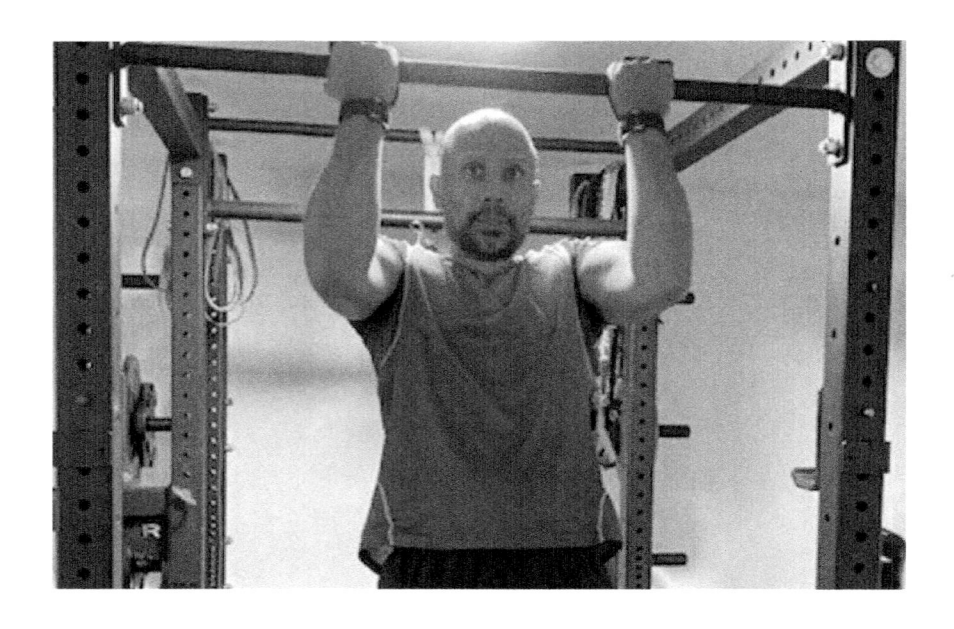

Ravi Strarup-Dhami was supposed to be a full-time computer expert – but he felt like he was in the army.

Working out seven days per week. Each training session dragged on and would last over 90 minutes. Constantly counting out the grams of protein, carbs and fat in every meal and writing everything down in his nutrition diary.

More like a torture camp than a fitness camp. Meanwhile, this was on top of trying to find time for his wife and kids too.

When 54-year-old Ravi first got into fitness 15 years ago, he didn't think it would have eventually led him to such a gruelling, military-style approach to training.

The Scotsman, who now lives in Germany, said: "I got into fitness was because I was overweight, lacking energy, I always felt tired, and I was fed up with the way I looked. This was due to a bad diet, eating crap takeaway foods, and drinking alcohol every weekend.

"I had joined my first gym back in Glasgow 30 years ago. Back then I was only doing cardio workouts, such as using the treadmill, rowing machines, and doing a few aerobic classes.

"I started to take my fitness serious again 15 years ago and built myself a home gym. I read about weight training online and started to incorporate it into my workouts. My goal then was to be muscular with a six pack. It never happened."

In chasing his fitness goals, Ravi signed up for seven different online fitness programs with big name coaches. He tried one after the other, hoping to find an effective system that would deliver results – and would fit in with his busy lifestyle as a father, husband and job as an IT systems engineer.

"I joined various online personal coaching programs and have not stopped since," said Ravi. "The main reason for leaving the other coaching methods behind is that I got tired from working out seven days a week.

"It felt as if I was in the army, and I never got much interaction from my online coach. I also got bored in counting my macronutrients every day and filling in my nutrition diary.

"These other online programs were just not family friendly."

Having first began his fitness journey doing cardio training, Ravi turned his attentions to weight training 15 years ago bumping into an old work colleague.

He had always remembered his old workmate as being very skinny, but was shocked and amazed to see how muscular the guy had become through dedicating himself to lifting weights.

That chance meeting gave Ravi inspiration and kick-started his new health hobby, however it took many failed approaches before he came across Be Your Own PT, and he signed up for the group coaching program in January 2020.

"I'm delighted I did. My workout programs from the other online coaches were to train seven days a week," said Ravi. "Doing compound and isolation movements for five sets and 8-10 reps. My workouts lasted over 90 mins.

"I like to try different approaches and the Be Your Own PT program approach was very simplistic, which caught my eye."

If ever there was a star pupil award it would go to Ravi. But he's a guy in his 50s – so that would be a bit weird. But seriously, Ravi is the type of guy to just do whatever is put in front of him and give 100%.

No delays, no looking for shortcuts, no messing around. Just putting in the work and doing what needs to be done.

I would set small weekly challenges for the group, such as directing them to send me pictures of a home-cooked healthy meal. Ravi's pictures would always arrive first.

On the program, each group member also submits their completed gym training diaries and a short weekly review to me at the end of the week. Some people would be late, some would forget. Ravi's was always submitted first and completed with care and attention.

It demonstrated focus, continued motivation, and it kept him firmly on track. This accountability tactic also showed in Ravi's progress throughout the program. Week by week he was lifting more weights, doing more repetitions, and getting particularly good at exercises he struggled with.

Muscle, Strength...And Chin-Ups

When he first signed up to Be Your Own PT, I asked Ravi: "What are the top three things you want to achieve through this 10-week fitness program?"

He replied: "Build muscle, become strong...and to do chin-ups."

All three goals have been achieved, and he over-achieved with chin-ups. By around week 7, he was so strong at chin-ups that I asked Ravi to use a dip belt and strap weights to his waist to make it even more difficult.

By week 10, Ravi was doing chin-ups while carrying 11lbs strapped to his waist, and managed 16 reps over three sets in his final workout.

Not bad for a guy just doing three training sessions per week, not seven. Pretty good for a guy doing 50-60 mins workouts, not ones that last over 90 mins. And some damn fine progress for a guy following a simpler diet – and not feeling like he's an army recruit any longer.

Ravi said:"I have more energy, my strength has increased considerably, and better muscle definition. The nutrition side of things is easy to follow, as is working out three days a week.

"You don't need a complicated program to achieve your goals. Stop counting calories – and learn about intermittent fasting instead.

"I also learned to stop being negative when training, such as thinking 'I'll not be able to lift this', or 'I won't be able to do any pull ups'. I overcame this by believing in myself, being positive, and just enjoying the workout.

"I'm still amazed at how much strength I gained over the 10 weeks. I'll continue following this training method now. In fact, I've not stopped training after I completed the 10 weeks. I've cleared the weekly workout sheets and just started again."

Chapter 18

Weight Training Has Got Me Back On Track

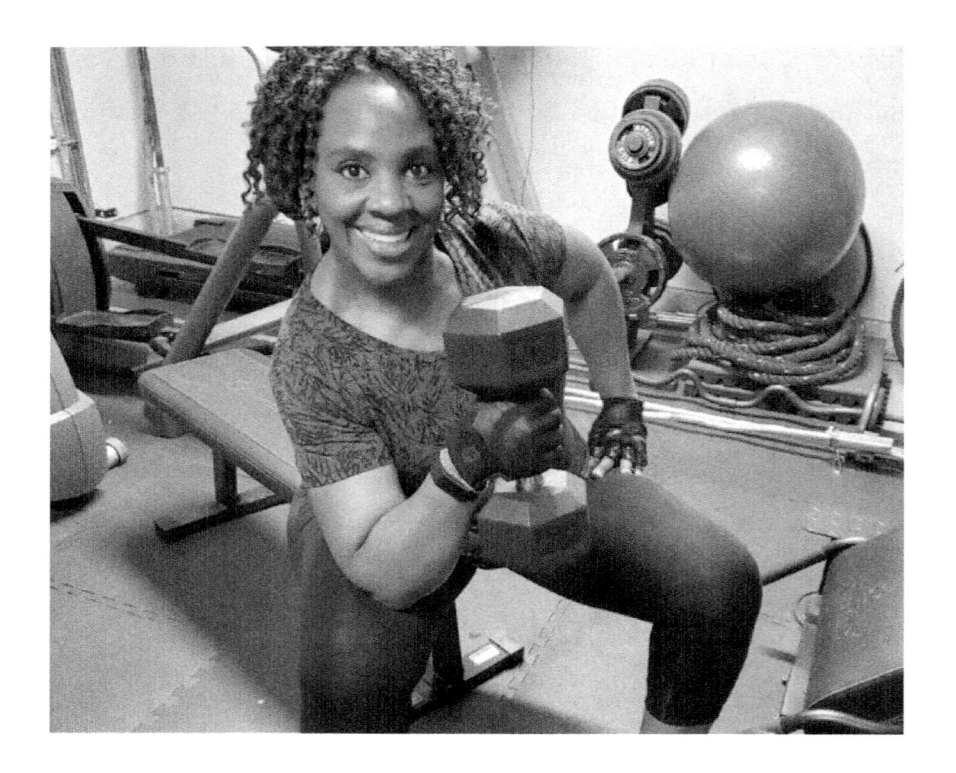

Dropped 100lbs back in 2010. Picked up weight training a couple of years later. Fitness and life in general had been going perfectly for Dorothea Mohan…

Until 2015 came around.

Disaster struck after the California mum-of-three had a surgical procedure, which put everything on hold.

"From 2012-2015 life seemed perfect, and my weight training was on point," said Dorothea. "In mid-2015 I had a hysterectomy that seemed to roadblock everything. Everything changed, I struggled daily, weekly, yearly to get back to where I was before my surgery.

"Nothing seemed to inspire or motivate me as I felt I was slipping into depression."

Dorothea was doing well in her career in banking and was happily married to Roger with three kids, but health and fitness had become a real struggle following the hysterectomy.

"I've always struggled with my weight, but I was always interested in doing something about it and getting fit," said Dorothea. "In 2010 I changed my lifestyle for good and embarked on a new journey. I had rededicated myself to health and fitness, and I've always loved how working out made me feel."

In 2016, Dorothea was searching for guidance after regaining some weight. There were so many tireless attempts at different exercise programs, taking weight loss pills, and following restricted diet plans. They all fell short of Dorothea's expectations.

The exercise programs were uninspiring. The restrictive meal plans were a chore. It was no wonder Dorothea quickly lost interest in each of them as there were no tangible results or benefits, but that didn't mean she was quitting.

Having already read my Strength Training For Women book, Dorothea knew she was on the right track with weight training as her fitness weapon on choice. She just needed an effective, manageable program.

That's exactly why she signed up with the others to the Be Your Own PT group coaching program.

"Ten weeks was the shortest program I had come across, and I felt that it was doable," said Dorothea.

"The structure of the weight training program, the one on one support, and the exercise video aids were the most helpful things for me."

It was clear to see after just a few weeks that Dorothea wouldn't be giving up on this fitness program. She was sharing positive feedback with me and other group members about loving her workouts, and making progress on various exercises.

As she began to score excellent personal bests in her workouts, the love for training and confidence in herself returned. One area I felt that was holding Dorothea back was her big focus on weight loss and the added pressure she was putting on her shoulders by weighing herself every day.

In general, I'm not a fan of people using the scales at all. As mentioned earlier, they are not the only marker of fitness progress — and constantly dwelling on weights numbers can create mental blocks which hinder progress overall.

This is something I chatted with Dorothea about halfway through the program as it was clearly holding her back, and making her fitness journey less enjoyable.

"I'm such a visual person when it comes to my weight loss because of where I've been," said Dorothea. "It was burdening me and in a sense I was sabotaging myself by doing this.

"Having the added group support proved to be an asset! Being able to talk to others on the same journey as me, men and women, made the vision so much clearer. I felt that I was going to hold myself accountable — but the other people plus Marc would see to it that I did!

"The program has left me in the right frame of mind to continue on my journey. I'm taking it day by day and will continue to train three days a week — and of course always accomplish PBs!"

Chapter 19

I Wanted To Be A Fitter And Healthier Dad

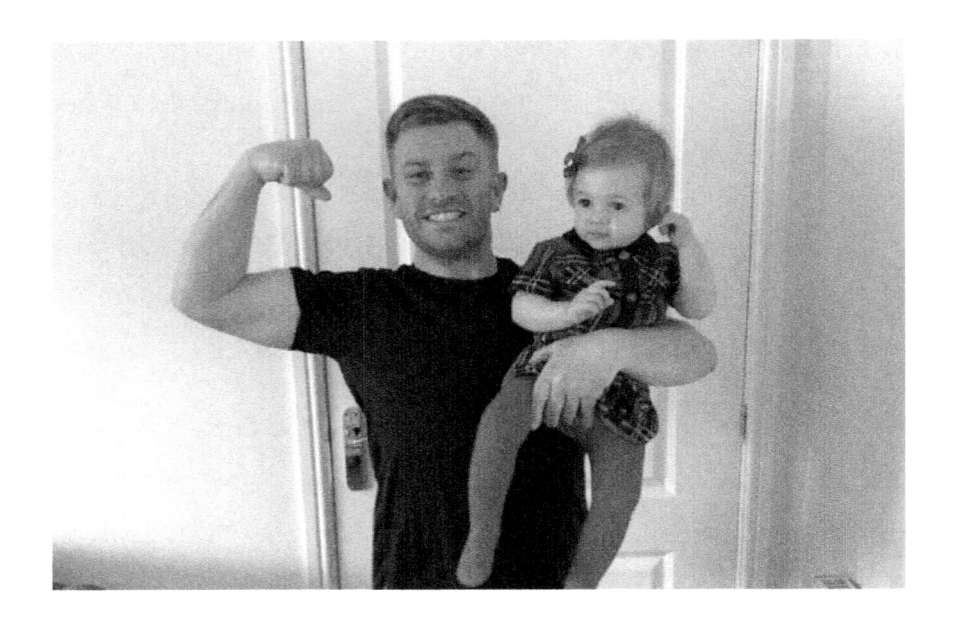

As Johnny looked down and saw the numbers staring back at him, he couldn't believe he'd allowed things to get so bad again.

It was November 2019 and it was the first time he'd stepped onto the scales to check his weight for a while.

What a difference a year makes. Because in November 2018, life was completely different. Johnny had lost 26lbs by that point through weight training and eating more sensibly, and was feeling fantastic as he holidayed in Cancun, Mexico, with his fiancée Danielle.

Back then, he was looking great, fit and strong, and it was the first holiday in a while where he was comfortable and wearing normal sized clothes instead of huge XL t-shirts.

All that was a distant memory as he peered down at the scales in the bathroom and the numbers 216.4 glared back at him. 216lbs – the heaviest he'd ever been in his life – and as he's not the tallest of guys, it put him firmly in the obese category.

"I was disgusted that I had allowed it to get to that point," said 34-year-old Johnny. "Especially after I had done so well with the weight training program first time around."

This is the point where readers will fully appreciate the honesty of people like Johnny, and many will relate to what he's gone through. Why? Because many men and women do well on training programs or specific diet plans, make great progress, and then lose it all again.

That's one of the main reasons I wanted to share Johnny's story in this book – for authenticity and to examine why things go wrong so that you can avoid the same mistakes.

Johnny and I grew up in the same area in the West of Scotland. He's a couple of years younger than me and our front doors were about 100 yards apart.

We lived in the same town as adults too, but didn't see each other very often. Then in 2018, I got an unexpected private Facebook message from Johnny pleading with me to help him lose fat, gain muscle and get in decent shape.

"I've tried everything, worked hard for months, and I've barely lost a single pound," he told me.

Long story short, Johnny did the very program I've laid out for you earlier in this book and dropped 26lbs in 10 weeks. He was hooked on the intermittent fasting + weight training + accountability approach, and jetted off on the holiday to Cancun a very happy man.

So, what went wrong? How did he manage to regain all that weight – and a bit more?

Life took an unexpected twist – on two fronts. He became a dad to a beautiful girl called Emily, and work became increasingly busy.

Lack of sleep at home. Stress at work. Upheaval. Feeling uptight. Life disorganisation. These were all key factors that led to workouts being skipped, eating junk food on the go, boozing a bit more, and generally not looking after himself properly.

"I was making too many excuses and I had slipped back into old habits," said Johnny. "But I knew this program worked – as I'd done it before.

"My daughter Emily was then eight months old by the time I had reached 216lbs again and I wanted to be fit and healthy so I could be the best dad and have more energy and time for her and my family.

"I was even more determined to get focused on the weight training and fasting again, and this time I was going to do even better than before."

For his situation to change, Johnny obviously had to change. And to avoid a yo-yo situation where his weight was up and down, he had to implement new daily habits – and adopt a new lifestyle.

What did that mean? Firstly, he had to *make* time for fitness. Anyone who says they can't find time for three one-hour gym workouts per week is simply bullshitting themselves. There are 168 hours per week, and you're awake for roughly 112 of them.

Dedicate just three of those hours to weight training and, if you work long hours, then get out of bed an hour earlier, and drag your ass to the gym. You'll be surprised at how much more energy you have for the rest of your day and how productive you are when you've started it strongly with a good weights session.

That's what Johnny did. Since he usually left for work at 6.45am, he was in the gym for 5.30am three days per week. After pushing himself hard in the mornings, he was flying on the post-workout endorphins and was able to handle the stress of his construction site job so much better.

No more losing his temper with workmates, getting pissed off at company bosses, or simply meeting work requirements. Instead, he was getting jobs completed more efficiently, leading his team of young tradesmen better, and going home at the end of the day feeling in control, rather than mentally and emotionally zapped.

With weekly workouts in check, Johnny also had to implement and maintain new dietary habits. Of course, that meant returning to intermittent fasting five days per week, and he also chose to track his food intake via the MyFitnesspal app.

Food tracking is not totally necessary as I believe you quickly grasp roughly how many calories, protein etc is in your meals each day, but Johnny was laser-focused on his goal and relied on using the app for peace of mind.

It was also necessary that Johnny reduce the chocolate biscuits, the crisps, and other junk food items in his diet that had led to piling weight back on again. This was tackled directly with the positive habits in various weeks of the program.

What was also important on the diet front was preparing food in the evenings. That meant cooking healthy meals at home, preparing lunch for the next day, making a healthy shake at night and grabbing it on the way to work in the morning. All simple, but very important steps.

Leaner & Stronger Every Week

Back in the game and focused by the end of November, Johnny was hitting the gym hard and eating clean again – even through the Christmas period.

By the time I opened up my group coaching program in January 2020 and he got involved, Johnny already had a head start and had dropped from 216lbs to 205lbs. Still, he was fired up to make even more progress by the end of the 10 weeks.

Johnny's 'muscle memory' clearly kicked in because it wasn't long before Johnny was increasing his weight levels in the gym and pushing his body hard. (Muscle memory is a term used when your muscles quickly regain previous strength levels after a period of inaction).

Initially doing chin-ups, dips and pull-ups with assistance, Johnny was able to do these exercises without any assistance a few weeks down the line as his bodyweight dropped while his muscle strength increased. By the end of the program, he was doing dips with weights strapped to his waist with a belt.

Having already lost 11lbs with weight training again before join my group coaching, Johnny set himself a target of losing another 20lbs and reaching 185lbs – the same he weighed when he felt at his "best" the previous year.

It was all looking good. Hitting new milestones each week. People commenting on how much slimmer he looked; how they could even see it in his face. Dropping from size XL clothes to L, and then having to return the L t-shirts for M instead because they were too big and baggy for him.

Stepping on the scale at the end of the 10 weeks was going to be a proud moment.

"I couldn't believe it," said Johnny. "My weight was 177lbs and it's stayed around the same for weeks afterwards. During the 10-week program I lost 28lbs, and 39lbs in total after deciding to take up weight training again.

"It's not just the weight loss though, doing all of this has completely changed my mentality. I'm more focused and positive, and feel a lot more assertive.

"I think it's all down to the discipline with your workouts and diet, and looking after your health and fitness. That naturally makes you feel better about yourself, and you grow in confidence.

"I feel strong, I really enjoy the gym, and I like pushing myself physically – especially because I know how much it benefits me mentally.

"All of this hard work benefits you and it's for you. You're not doing it to please anyone else, it's to make yourself healthier, happier and for your life to run smoother.

"Some people get into fitness because they've got a holiday coming up. Or some of my mates will go to the gym because they're going on a stag do a couple of months down the line.

"That's not really what this should be all about. It should be about keeping this lifestyle going so that you're happier, healthier and have a better mindset overall."

That's all well and good – but what happens when coronavirus strikes and virtually every gym on the planet shuts down?

No sweat. Within a day of lockdown, Johnny had bought a home weights set and was working out in his garage. Being a strong and healthy dad is a priority these days.

"After Emily was born I reached the heaviest weight I'd ever been, and I was unhappy with myself at a time when I should have been at my happiest," said Johnny.

"I knew it was time to change and looking back on it now, I think 'how the hell did I allow that to happen to myself'?

"Weight training and looking after myself better is an important part of my routine now. I weigh myself once per week on a Saturday now, and diet-wise I just do what we do on the program — eat healthy Monday-Friday and have some treats at the weekend.

"I now have more energy and can spend better quality time with Emily and Danielle, and I have a completely different mentality. These have been the best benefits."

Bonus Chapter: Supplements

You've got the full gym membership, you're going to clean up your diet, and you're ready to train like a maniac for the next 10 weeks. Now what?

Will a healthy diet be enough for developing lean muscle and losing unwanted fat? Will your body respond perfectly, and everything magically fall into place?

You absolutely can achieve your fitness goals long term by working out hard, eating well, and ensuring you get sufficient rest. But here's where things get a little tricky.

Where we live in the Western world it's harder to take in enough of the essential vitamins and minerals every day with our standard diet. Even if you eat a lot of fruit and veg daily, it's not guaranteed that you'll be consuming enough nutrients due to issues like soils being depleted, produce being sprayed with chemicals etc.

Secondly, our lives can be pretty stressful at times working long hours, looking after the kids, money worries etc. This results in stress hormones being released and the body has to use up important minerals such as magnesium to deal with that – which can ultimately lead to deficiencies.

When you throw tough weight training workouts into the mix, there's a temporary physical stress on the body which also demands extra nutritional support. And of course, you should be doing everything you can to properly recover from those weights workouts.

You can see where I'm going with this. In order to stay healthy, strong, and give your body the tools it needs to develop in accordance with your fitness goals, then it's a very smart move to use some natural supplements.

Supplements For Strength, Health and Wellbeing

It's not necessary to spend a fortune on supplements, there are some really good ones out there that are reasonably priced. Also, I'm about to list six key supplements below that are always in my cupboards.

But please don't be overwhelmed by this – or think that you have to stock up on them all. I consider three of them to be essentials for best results, while the others are helpful...but only if you've got extra money to afford them.

Plant-Based Protein Powder (Essential)

Drinking a protein shake around an hour post-workout will provide your muscles with a good source of much-needed protein and a smaller amount of carbohydrates to kick-start the muscle repair and development process.

I switched from whey protein (dairy-based) to a plant-based alternative (made from pea, bean, brown rice etc) around six or seven years ago.

Many (not all) of the whey proteins on the market contain sweeteners, various additives, and the heat processing involved to extract the whey also makes it harder to digest.

If you then mix this whey powder with milk, which contains lactose (it's estimated that two thirds of adults are lactose intolerant), your digestive system is then going to have even more difficulty breaking down the shake.

Plant-based protein is easily digested and highly absorbable, meaning your muscles can soak up more of that protein for repair and development. Whatever type or brand you choose, your protein powder is best mixed with water.

* **My recommendations:** Vegan Blend from MyProtein.com or Warrior Blend from Sunwarrior.com.

Vitamin & Mineral Tablet (Essential)

The body uses vitamins and minerals to repair and replace cells. We simply cannot function properly without them. The standard

Western diet and processing of food strips what we eat of its goodness.

The result? Vitamin and mineral deficiencies. These deficiencies can cause various niggling health issues. For example, if you lack vitamin B12 you'll likely feel tired, out of breath, or develop headaches.

Taking a good vitamin and mineral supplement helps ensure you cover all bases, and is a wise investment for foundational health.

* **My recommendation:** Nature's Own food state multivitamins and minerals, which cost around $30 for a three-month supply on Amazon.com.

Zinc, Magnesium & Vitamin B6 Formulation, also known as 'ZMA' (Essential)

This is a tremendous and inexpensive vitamin and mineral supplement which is well used by people who lift weights who are clued-up about the importance of the recovery process. It's a post-workout essential in my view, and I take ZMA around one hour before bed.

This combination of two minerals (zinc and magnesium) and one vitamin (B6) is a potent mix for recovery and growth because it assists in hormone production and a deep, restful sleep.

Training hard in the gym consistently can lower levels of testosterone, as can everyday life stresses, but this supplement has been clinically proven to increase anabolic hormone levels and muscle strength in athletes.

* My recommendation: Optimum Nutrition ZMA capsules, which can usually be bought on Amazon.com or found on other sports nutrition websites via a Google search.

Creatine Monohydrate (Helpful)

This is one pre-workout supplement recommended for people who are focused more on muscle and strength development, but not those primarily aiming for weight loss.

Creatine is a natural compound that enhances your body's production of adenosine triphosphate (ATP). In simple terms, ATP is the most basic form of energy in your body's cells.

Beef and salmon are among the best food sources of creatine – but you would have to eat silly amounts to get the levels you need. That's why, since 1993, creatine has become a popular supplement in powder/capsules for athletes.

More creatine = more ATP = you training harder and longer in the gym. Creatine also has various other benefits including fuller muscles as it draws more fluid into your muscles, enhanced recovery as reduces cell damage and inflammation, and better brain function.

Supplementing with creatine can result in a marked increase in your strength levels and help you perform even better in the gym.

Sports nutrition experts recommend that you take between 3g and 5g of creatine daily. It's also recommended that you take breaks in order to optimise its effectiveness. For example, I take creatine for two months on, and then one month off.

Don't exceed recommended amounts and always seek advice from a medical professional if you have any health queries or concerns.

* **My recommendation:** Optimum Nutrition creatine monohydrate capsules, also available via Amazon.com.

Magnesium Oil (Helpful)

This is a fantastic supplement for health and vitality, and can do wonders for your sleep if you struggle to get a decent night's rest.

The mineral magnesium plays such an important role in the healthy functioning of the body – yet it's been estimated that 75% of people living in Western society are deficient in magnesium.

This is because the stresses of 21st century living, poor diet, being overworked, lack of sleep etc deplete our levels of this miracle mineral.

Supplementing with magnesium oil is also beneficial for men and women lifting weights and other athletes because it relaxes and soothes sore muscles, speeding up recovery times following tough workouts.

It's also an amazing aid for a good night's sleep as it calms the nervous system by inhibiting cortisol and adrenaline (two major stress hormones). Proper sleep is so important to muscle development and overall health.

You could eat the healthiest diet possible filled with organic, wholesome foods...but it'd never make up for a lack of sleep in terms of maintaining good health.

Our hormones can also be thrown out of whack with the pressures of our job, relationship difficulties, and financial worries. This has a knock-on negative impact on your physical health.

Magnesium is a top tool for helping to balance your hormones – and it has an added calming effect when you are stressed.

I choose the oil rather than tablets because applying it to your skin results in more magnesium being absorbed by the body. For best results, spray 8-10 times on each arm and rub it in around one hour before bed. Then wipe off before going to sleep.

Give it around a week to feel the effects – as you may have been deficient in magnesium for a while.

*** My recommendation:** Ancient Minerals magnesium oil, which can be bought on Amazon.com.

Green Tea Extract (Helpful)

I'm listing green tea extract capsules/tablets as a healthier pre-workout alternative to energy drinks.

Way too many people rely on energy drinks for a boost in the gym, and mistakenly think these products are healthy because they apparently contain various vitamins and minerals.

You probably think: energy drink = caffeine boost = more energy = more fat burning.

Afraid not. The reality is: energy drink = artificial sweeteners + other unnatural ingredients = fat gain + potential health issues in the long term.

Sucralose is a common artificial sweetener in many of these drinks...and this is 600 X sweeter than sugar. Yes, 600.

Numerous studies have also linked artificial sweeteners to obesity and various other health problems.

Taking some green tea extract capsules before your workout with a tall glass of water is a much better idea. It's especially useful for people looking to lose weight – but always stick with the recommended dosage on the bottle.

Green tea extract contains caffeine, which will give you a welcome energy boost in the gym. Green tea is also rich in a key compound called epigallocatechin gallate, better known as EGCG, which is understood to reduce fat gain and increase fat burning.

You can't get a sufficient amount in a plain cup of green tea to experience these benefits, but green tea extract has EGCG in higher concentrations.

* **My recommendation:** MyProtein.com's own brand of green tea extract is a good choice and cheap to buy. Remember not to exceed the recommended daily dose as too much caffeine can interrupt your sleep and potentially tax your adrenals glands in the long term.

All six supplements I've listed are all-natural, safe, and free of any dodgy ingredients. I wouldn't recommend anything I haven't tried and tested for years myself.

Bottom line: these supplements will help you reach your fitness goals more quickly, and they'll assist in both your gym performances and the all-important recovery phase afterwards.

Conclusion

Strength. Confidence. Health.

These are the three most important areas of focus throughout Be Your Own PT. Forget bodybuilding, aesthetics, and the idea of trying to impress anyone else.

Your fitness story and your commitment to a 10-week program like this should be all about you…and becoming a stronger, more confident, healthier version of yourself.

That's the huge misconception with strength training. Too many people think that those who lift weights are egomaniacs obsessed with having the perfect body.

It's only when you dedicate yourself to a challenging, fairly-lengthy program like the one described in this book that you understand it's more about personal growth and improvement.

It's about being focused and driven in the gym – and then carrying those qualities into other area of your life.

And it's about developing self-worth and discipline through pushing yourself physically and mentally over an extended period of time.

Let's be clear: it isn't easy. If it is, you're not doing it right. Every gym session should be an opportunity for you to try and outdo your previous performance. It should always be challenging; no half-hearted workouts allowed.

And sometimes life gets in the way. I'm not going to pretend that every person who signs up to Be Your Own PT achieves huge success and wears a cape afterwards. No, there have been some drop-outs along the way due to family issues, health problems, and other unexpected situations.

That's to be expected. Some of the tough stuff life throws at us can knock us way off course. But my advice for anyone who has had to ditch workouts, or slipped into bad emotional eating habits again?

Drag your ass back to the gym and pick up some weights. Even if you're just going through the motions. Nine times out of 10 you'll feel completely different by the time you've finished your workout.

After taking that first step, writing yourself a plan of just three workouts for the week ahead – just like we do with Be Your Own PT – Monday, Wednesday, Friday. That plan will give you direction and focus, taking your mind off the negative crap that may be going on in your world.

Next step, make the commitment to a longer program. A 10-week one perhaps?

Where would you find one of those...all laid out for you...step by step? Yes, it's all there in Part Two of this book. Follow the 10-week program, and simply go through it week by week.

Copy the workout plans into a notepad, or your mobile phone notes app, and then follow along in the gym. Mark down the weights you've been lifting, how many repetitions, and keep track of everything.

Then you can set yourself targets to aim for, you can push for new personal bests, and build a rock-solid mindset while you develop a stronger, leaner body.

This stuff works. That's why I tried hard to convince the men and women in this book to share their stories with you. That was a gutsy move by them because we've all got our health and fitness hang-ups and insecurities, and it can be a little uncomfortable sharing your challenges and struggles with the world.

It was important for me to show you a selection of men and women that you can relate to, rather than the fitness model types with the perfect bodies and fake tan – just like I'd seen in that fitness book many years ago.

I want to empower you to take full charge of your fitness. The main aim of sharing the Be Your Own PT program in this book is to give you solid training/nutrition/accountability and mindset strategies that you can put into action – and finally see positive results from.

These are the same strategies I use every week. I've been using them for many years now, and I'm probably in better shape and healthier now at 37 than I was when I was 18.

You now have a solid plan for going forward, and it's not rocket science. Mainly compound exercises at first, more isolation exercises later, training 3 days per week, doing intermittent fasting Monday-Friday, hitting personal bests, and working on the mind game.

This stuff is not hard to maintain...you just need to keep taking action and stay consistent.

After the 10 weeks are over, why not go back to the start and do it all over? You'll be starting from an advanced level and will be able to move on up a gear with your training.

That's why I'm confident you can *Be Your Own PT*. Take control of your own health and fitness, but always remember to warm up well, and put good technique and safety first during your workouts.

This book provides a focused 10-week structured program to give you direction, accountability, and a solid foundation for staying fit and strong.

But what I want most for you is for this: those three weight training sessions per week, the intermittent fasting, and accountability tactics, to become a *healthy lifestyle that you maintain.*

About The Author

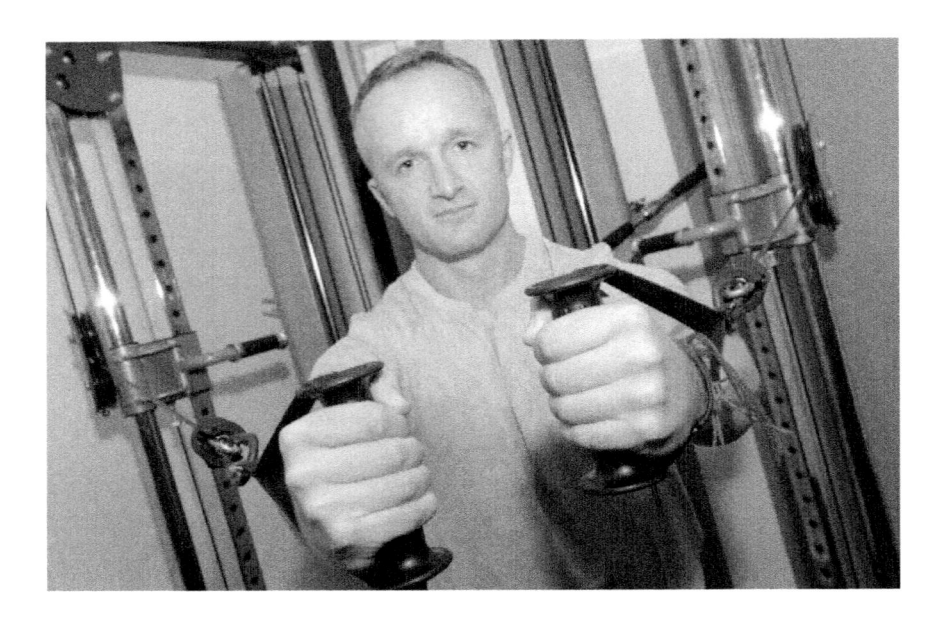

Weight training came first for Marc McLean at the age of 16. Writing came next when he began working as a journalist at his local newspaper three years later.

The gym hobby/obsession has never stopped in the past 22 years, and in 2015 Marc combined his two passions by launching his 'Weight Training Is The Way' blog in 2015.

The Scotsman became a fitness writer for leading websites Mind Body Green and The Good Men Project…and published the first in a series of weight training books in 2017.

EXERCISES INDEX

All the weight training moves included in the Be Your Own PT program

ARNIE PRESS (Works shoulders)

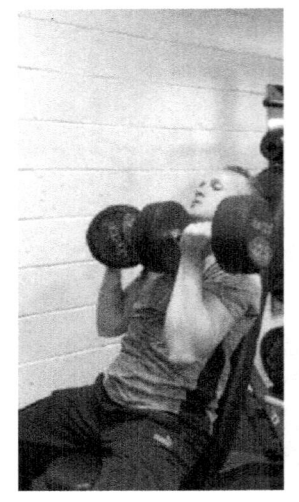

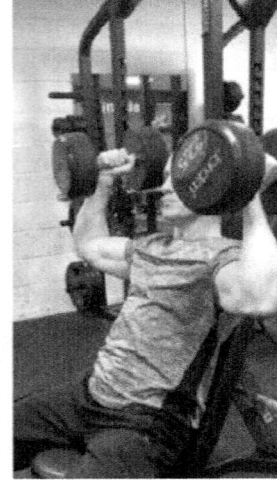

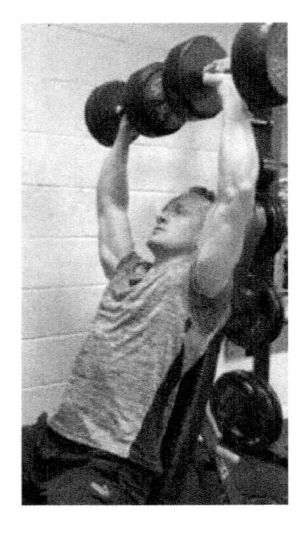

BARBELL CURLS (Works biceps, forearms)

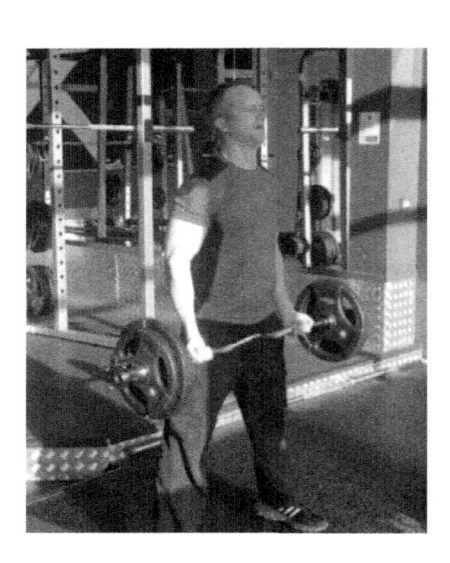

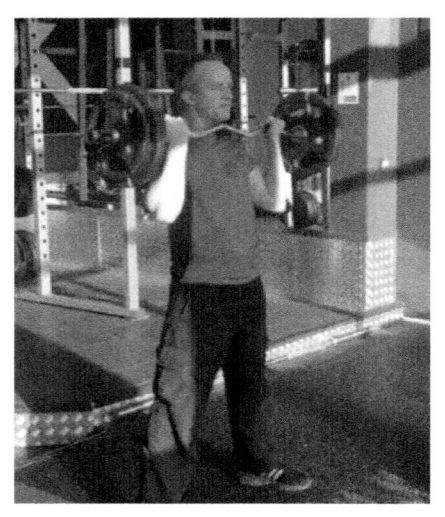

BENCH PRESS (Chest, shoulders, triceps)

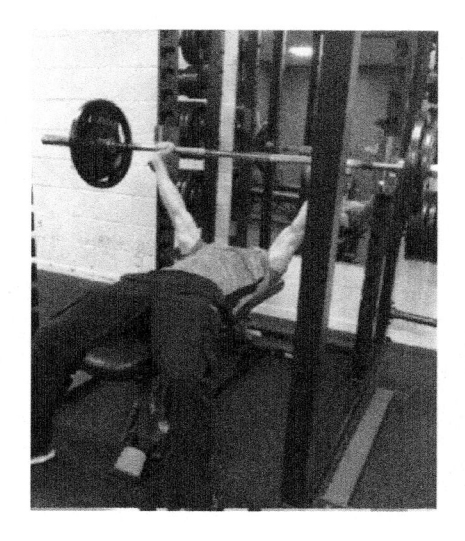

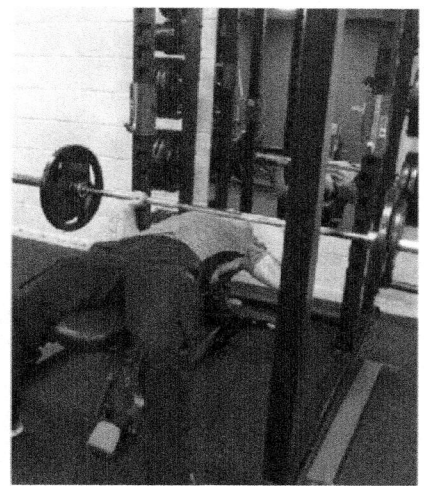

BENT OVER ROW (Latissimus dorsi 'lats', trapezius, biceps, shoulders, forearms)

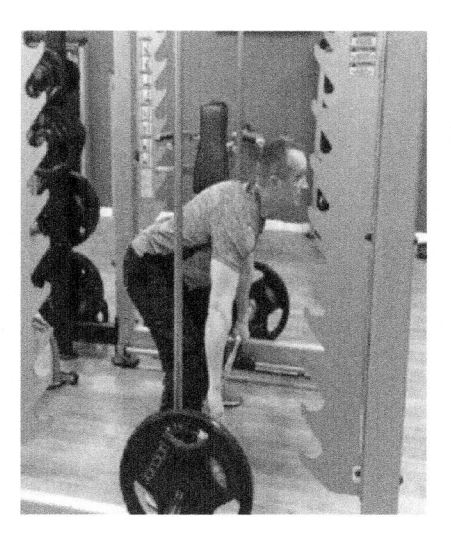

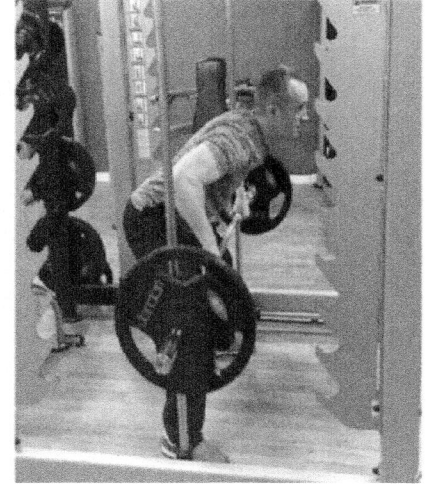

CABLE ROW (Lats, biceps)

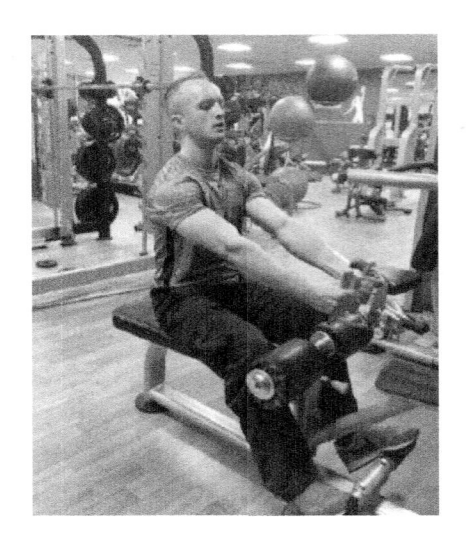

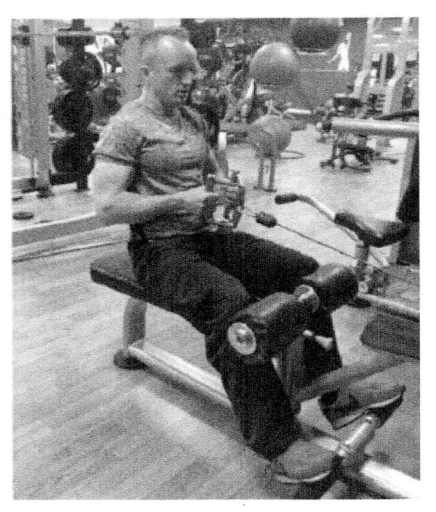

CHIN-UPS (Shoulders, biceps, lats, core, forearms)

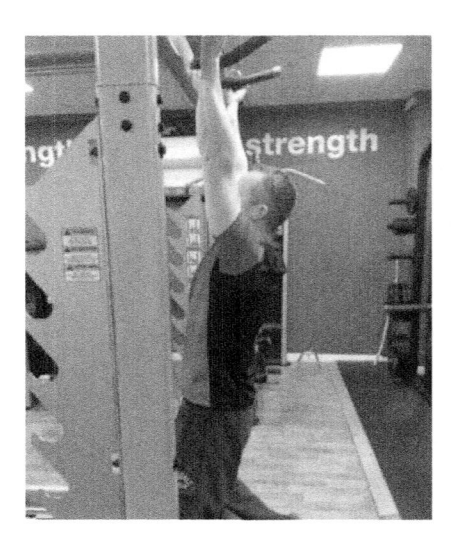

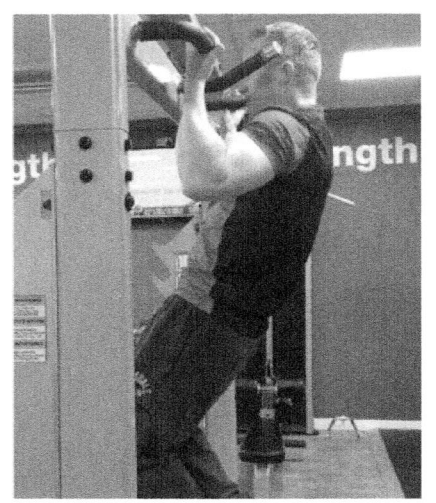

CLEAN & PRESS (Glutes, quadriceps, hamstrings, trapezius, shoulders, triceps, forearms)

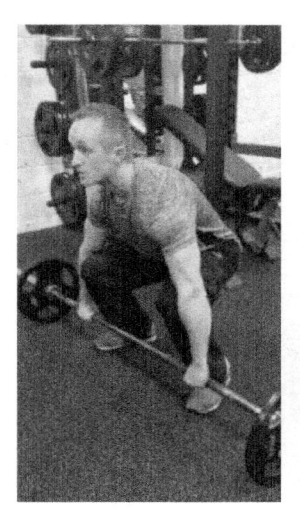

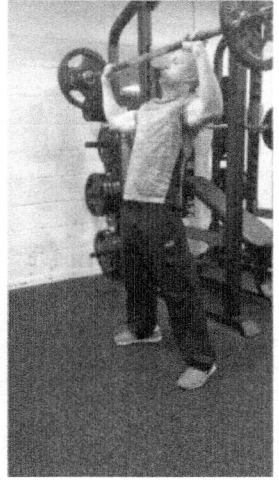

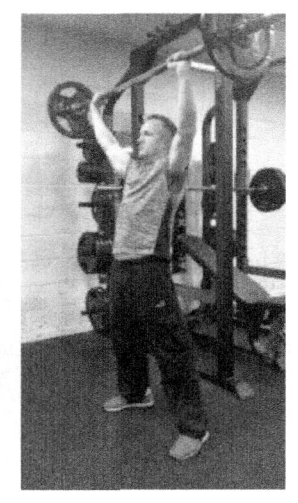

DEADLIFTS (Glutes, quadriceps, hamstrings, calves, lower back, core, shoulders, trapezius)

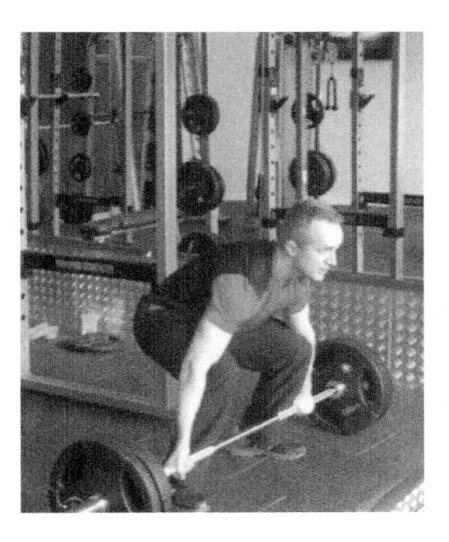

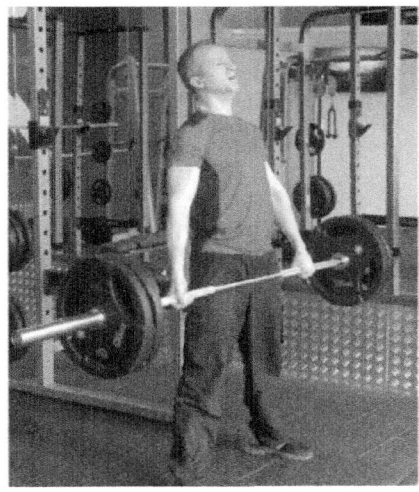

DELTOID RAISES (Shoulders)

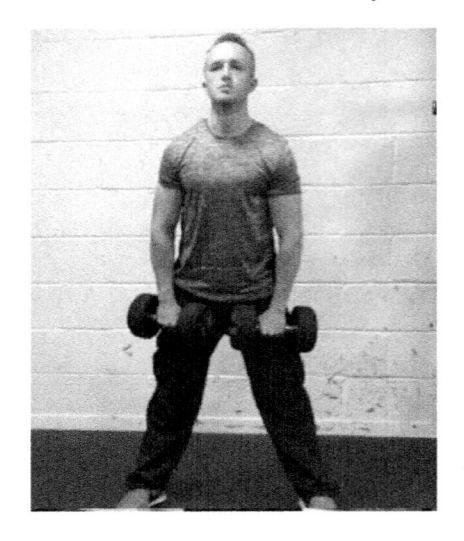

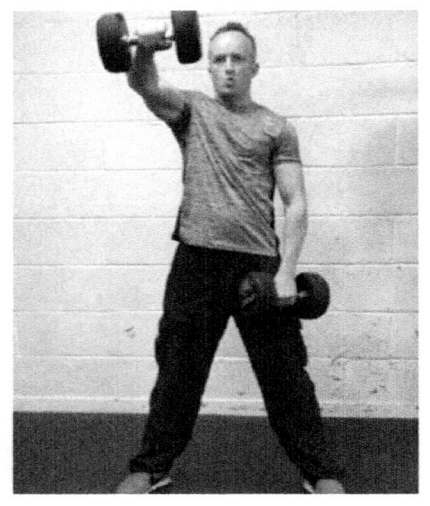

DIPS (Triceps, shoulders, chest, core)

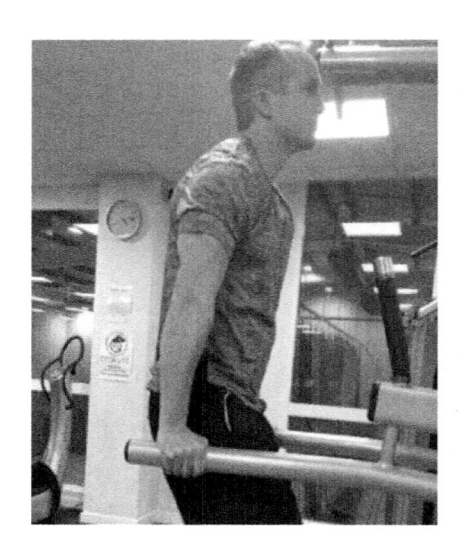

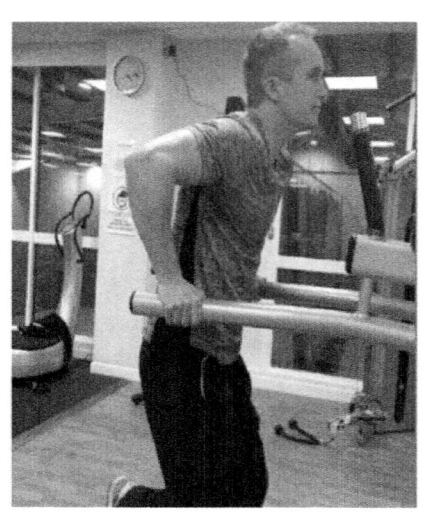

DUMBBELL FLYES (Chest, shoulders)

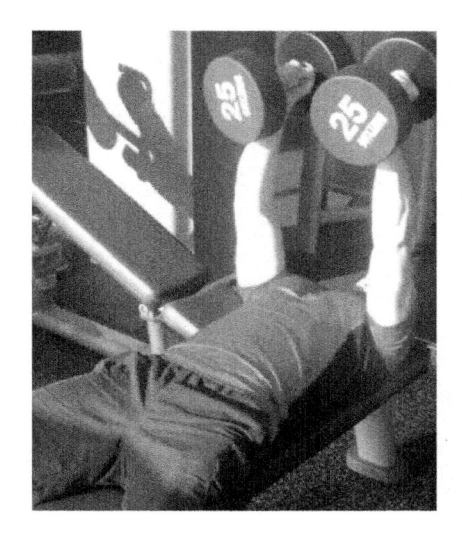

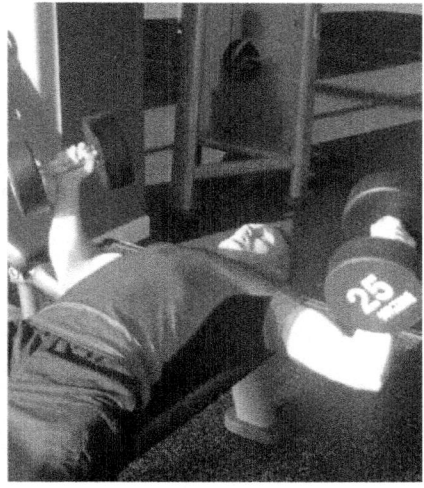

DUMBBELL PRESS (Chest, shoulders)

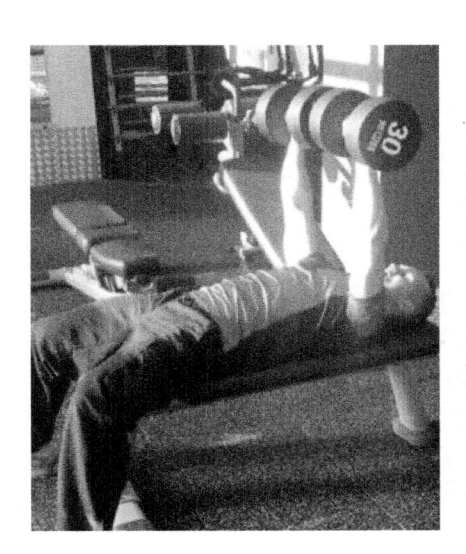

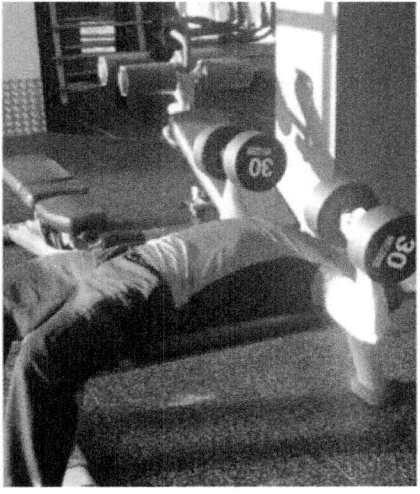

DUMBBELL LUNGES (Glutes, quadriceps, hamstrings, calves)

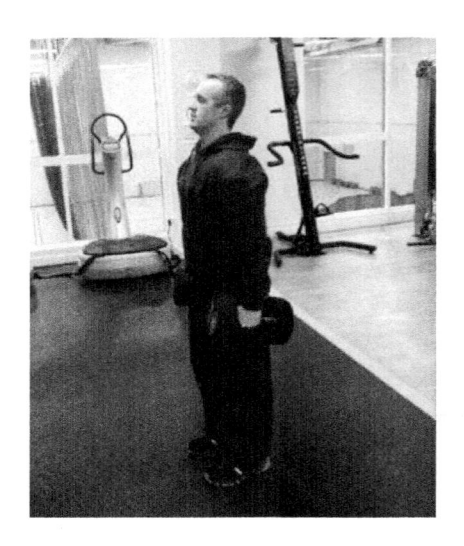

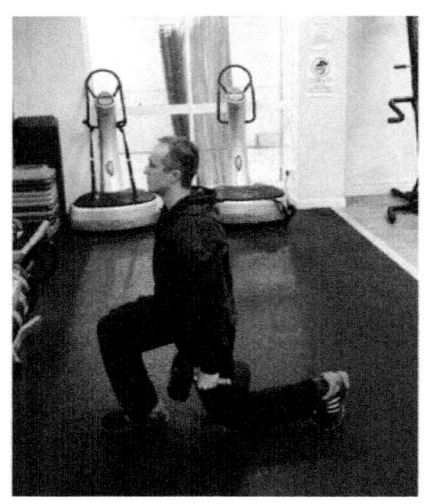

DUMBBELL ROW (Lats, biceps)

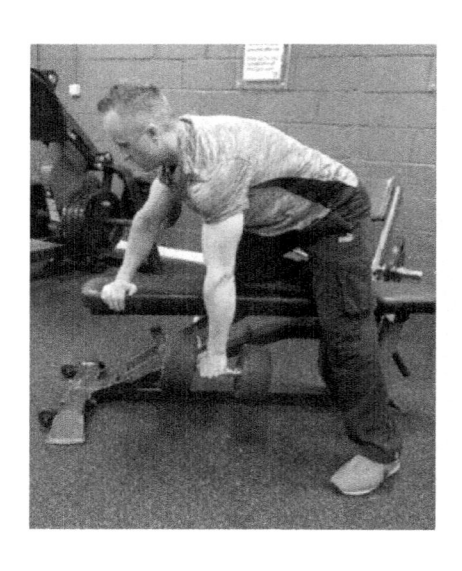

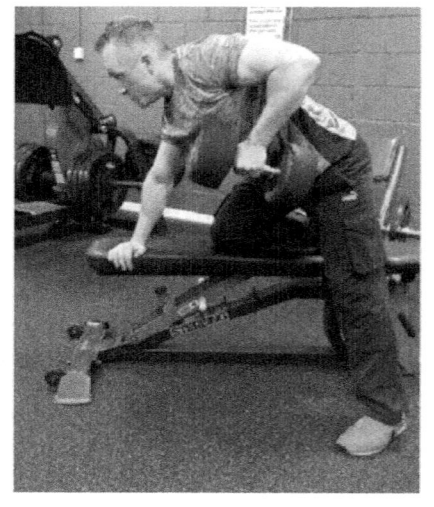

HAMSTRING MACHINE (Hamstrings)

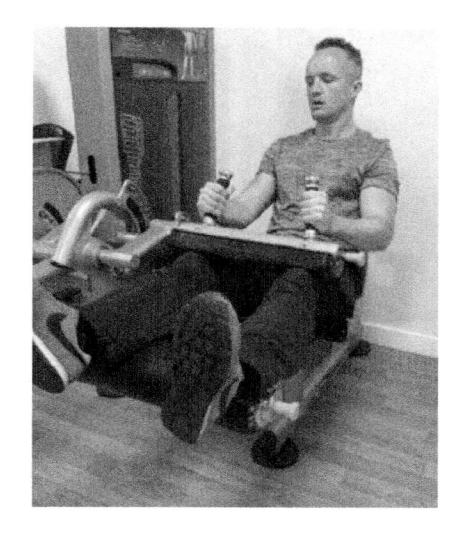

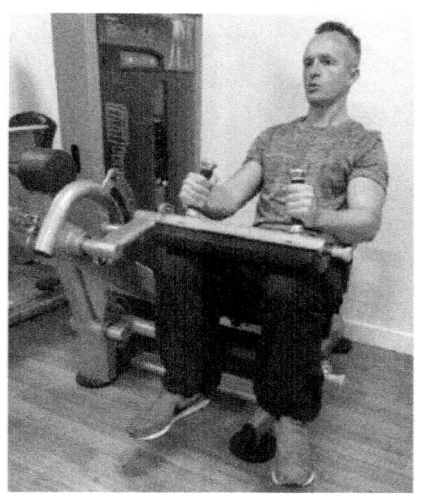

LAT PULLDOWN (Lats, shoulders, biceps)

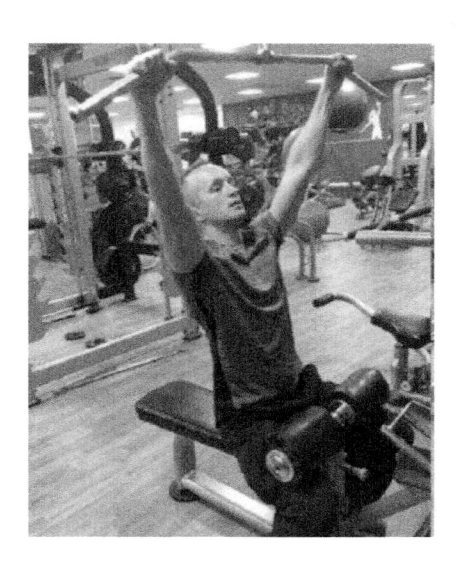

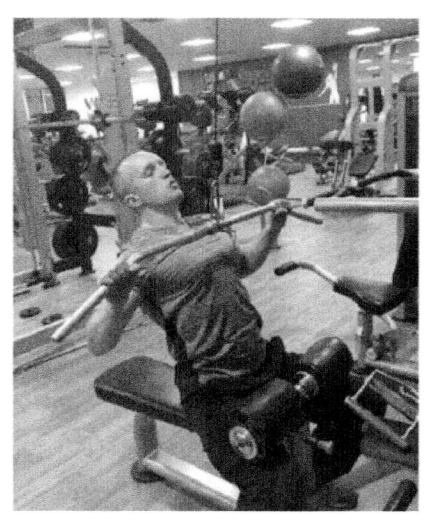

LYING BENCH CURLS (Biceps)

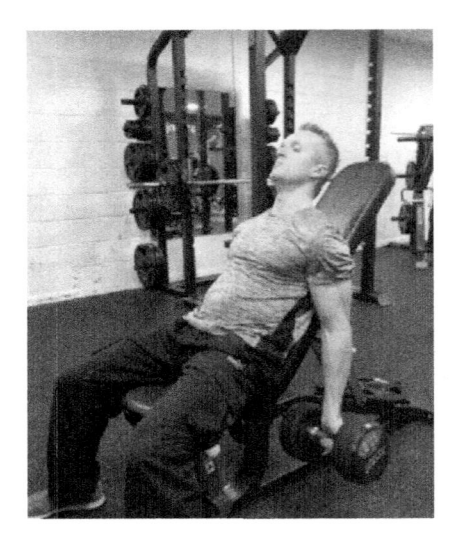

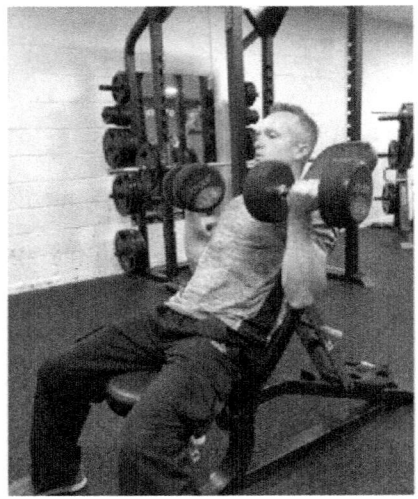

MILITARY PRESS (Shoulders, trapezius, arms)

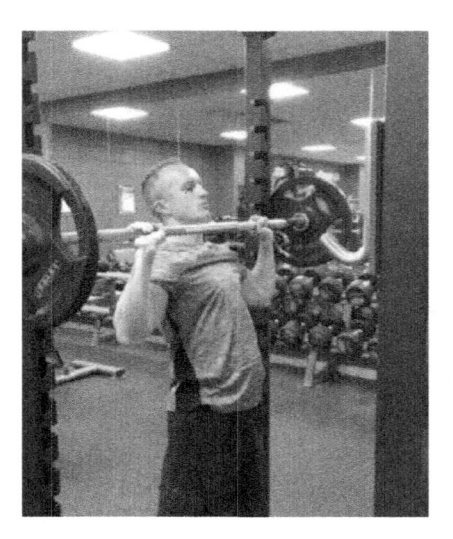

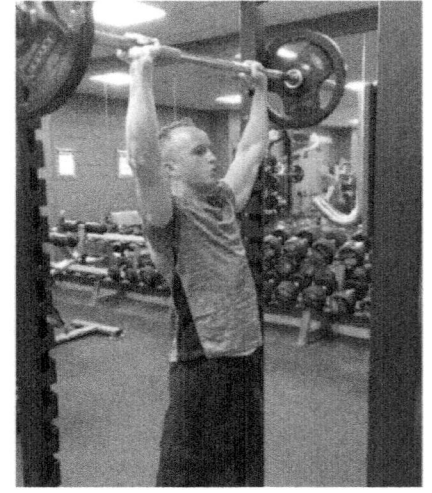

NARROW GRIP BENCH PRESS (Triceps)

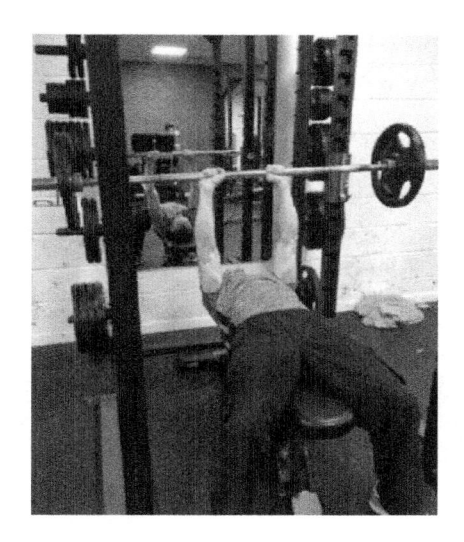

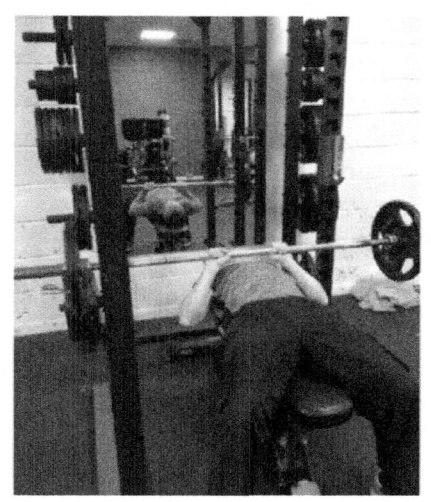

OVERHEAD ROPE EXTENSION (Triceps)

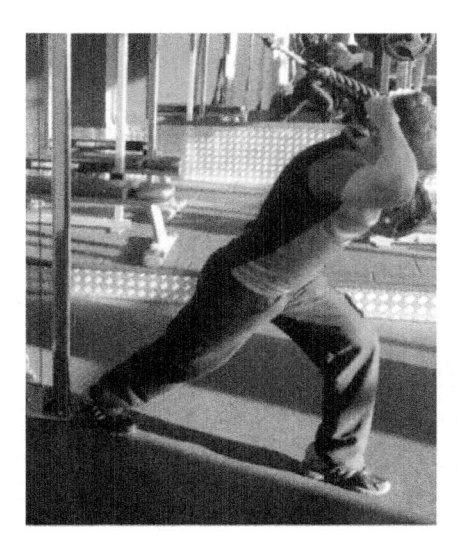

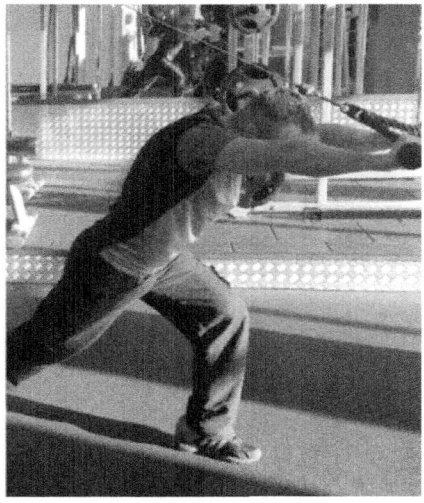

PULL-UPS (Lats, shoulders, trapezius, triceps, forearms, core)

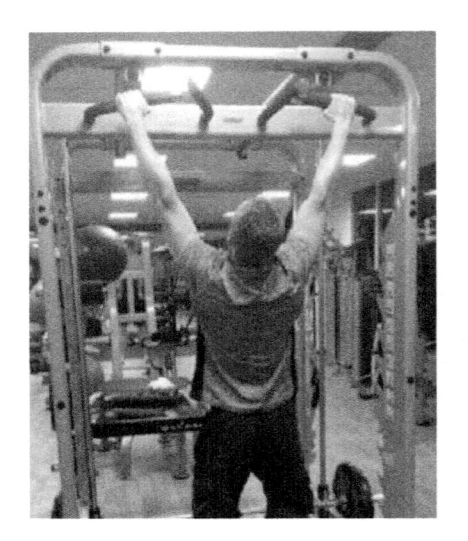

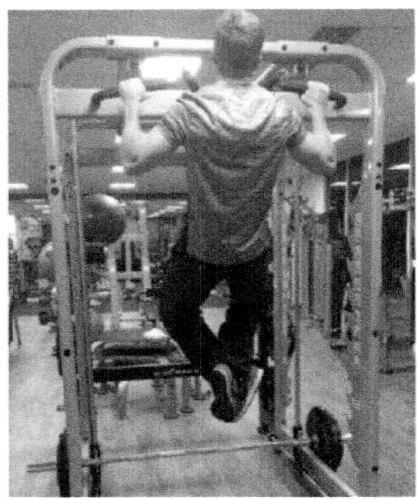

PEC DECK (Chest, shoulders)

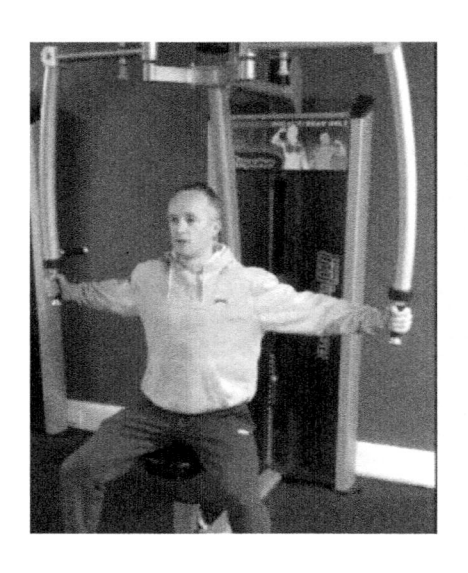

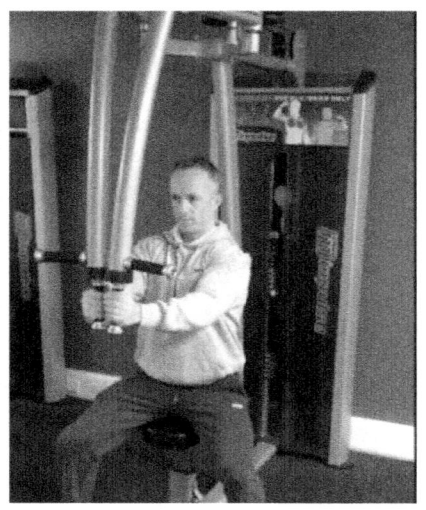

QUAD MACHINE (Quadriceps)

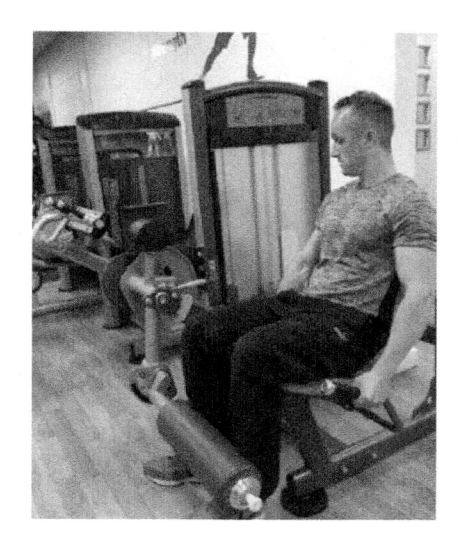

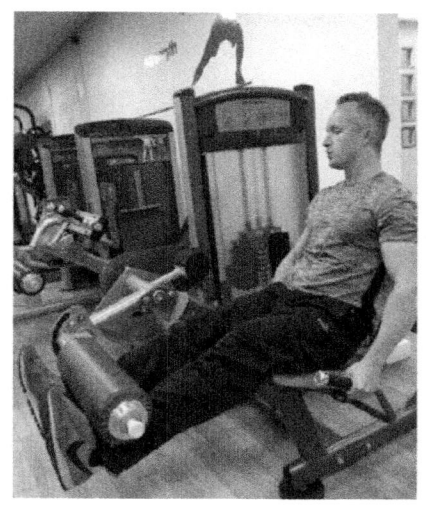

REVERSE FLYES (Shoulders, rear)

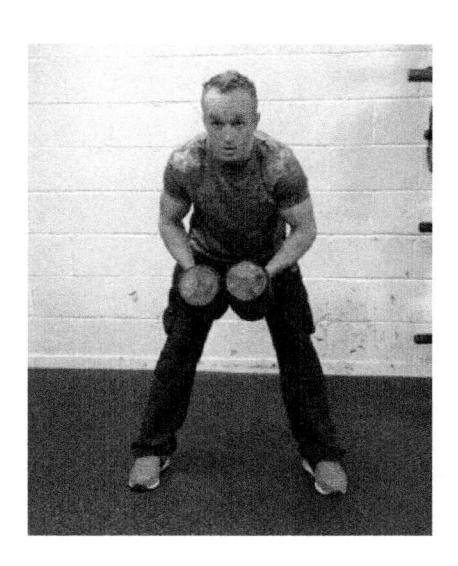

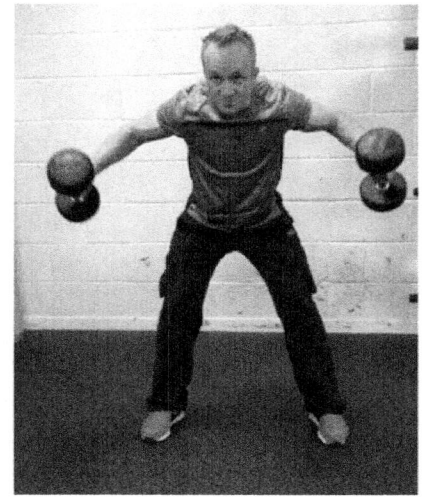

SQUATS (Glutes, quadriceps, hamstrings, calves, lower back, core)

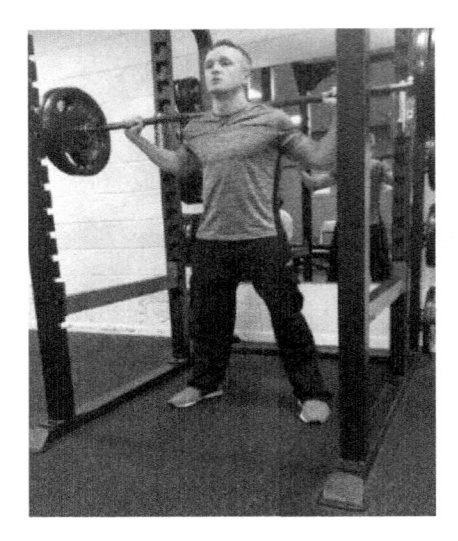

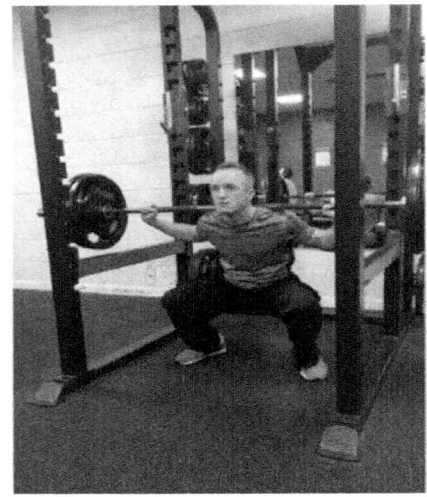

TRICEPS PUSHDOWN (Triceps)

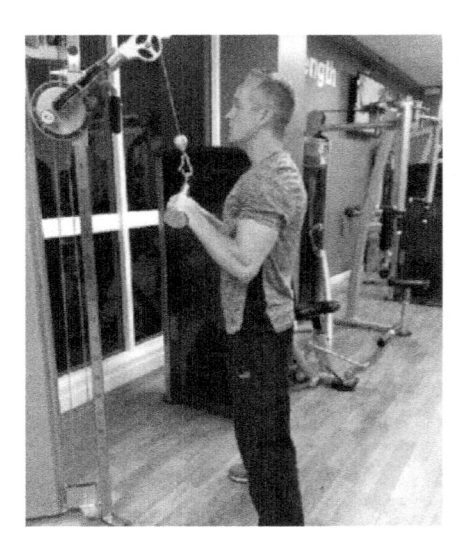

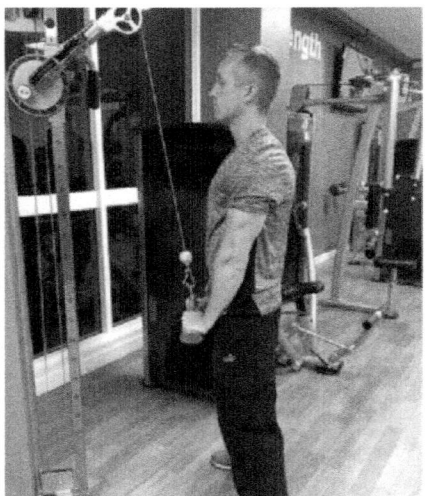

UPRIGHT ROW (Trapezius, biceps, shoulders, forearms)

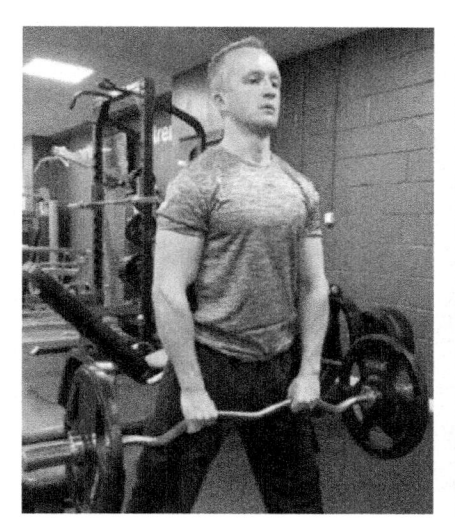

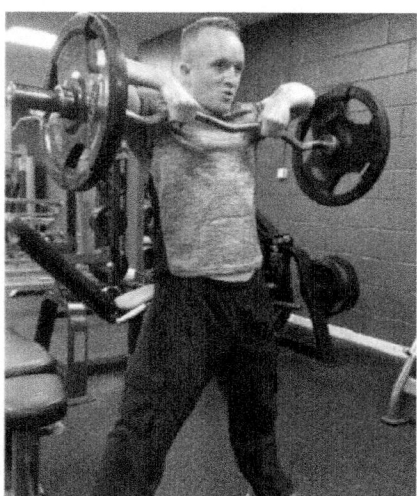

VIDEO DEMOS

Remember, there are also short video demo clips of every exercise included in this book on the Weight Training Is The Way YouTube channel:

http://www.youtube.com/c/WeightTrainingIsTheWay

BODYWEIGHT EXERCISES

The bodyweight exercises — chin-ups, pull-ups, and dips — are difficult to master at first. However, you can use assistance machines in the gym or resistance bands to give you added support until you develop enough upper body strength to do proper, unassisted repetitions.

I created a chin-ups video that helps guide you through this. You can view it here: https://youtu.be/JrA1MLfVo0c

Printed in Great Britain
by Amazon